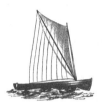

RARITAN SKIFF BOOKS

EDITED BY
JACKSON LEARS
AND
KAREN PARKER LEARS

RARITAN SKIFF BOOKS
IS A COLLABORATION BETWEEN
RARITAN QUARTERLY
AND
RUTGERS UNIVERSITY PRESS

PANDEMONIUM LOGS

◆

SIOUX FALLS, SOUTH DAKOTA

2020–2022

BEN MILLER

RARITAN SKIFF BOOKS

PUBLISHED BY RUTGERS UNIVERSITY PRESS

New Brunswick, Camden, and Newark, New Jersey

London and Oxford

Rutgers University Press is a department of Rutgers, The State
University of New Jersey, one of the leading public research
universities in the nation. By publishing worldwide, it furthers
the University's mission of dedication to excellence
in teaching, scholarship, research, and clinical care.

Library of Congress Cataloging-in-Publication Data

Names: Miller, Ben (Ben P.), author.
Title: Pandemonium logs : Sioux Falls, South Dakota 2020–2022 / Ben Miller.
Description: New Brunswick, New Jersey : Rutgers University Press, [2025] |
Series: Raritan Skiff Books
Identifiers: LCCN 2024012423 | ISBN 9781978835276 (paperback) |
ISBN 9781978835283 (hardcover) | ISBN 9781978835290 (epub) |
ISBN 9781978835306 (mobi) | ISBN 9781978835313 (pdf)
Subjects: LCSH: COVID-19 Pandemic, 2020—South Dakota—Sioux Falls. |
Miller, Ben (Ben P.) | Medical personnel—South Dakota—Sioux
Falls—Biography.
Classification: LCC RA644.C67 M5443 2025 | DDC 616.2/41440092
[B]—dc23/eng/20240613
LC record available at https://lccn.loc.gov/2024012423

A British Cataloging-in-Publication record for this
book is available from the British Library.

♾ The paper used in this publication meets the requirements of the
American National Standard for Information Sciences—Permanence
of Paper for Printed Library Materials,
ANSI Z39.48-1992.

rutgersuniversitypress.org

For Anne Pierson Wiese,
        a steadfast lyrical partner

And in memory of Agustín Rodríguez,
        Dr. Julie Butler,
        Tom Settle,
        and Cirino Zappala

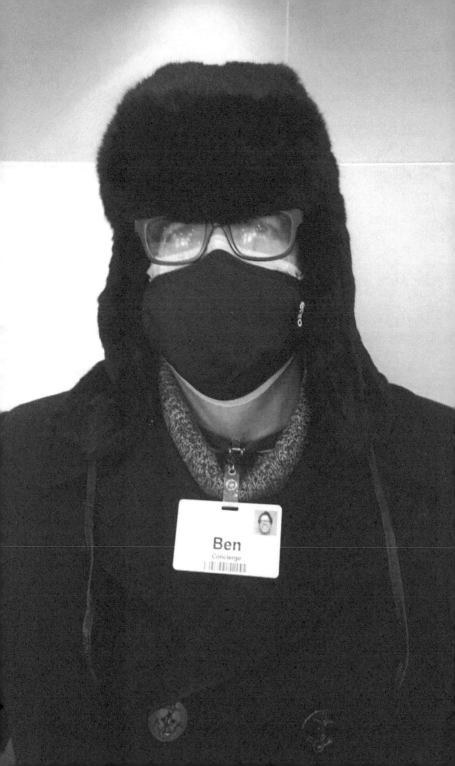

CONTENTS

PANDEMONIUM
LOGS

LOG 1

Call of the Killdeer

The dark depths of the Word numb me and immunize
me. I don't participate in the enchanting agony. With a
stone-like sobriety I remain the mother of distant cradles.
                                              —René Char, *Leaves of Hypnos*
                                              (trans. Cid Corman)

March 10–23, 2020
Scribe in Scrubs

Perpetuating the writer's existence required—in my case—a
clerk's life also be enacted. This spring it meant pulling three
twelve-hour shifts a week as a support specialist in a diminutive
(two doctor, two nurse) around-the-clock telehealth intensive
care unit that assists the ICU staff at thirty-four hospitals in a
territory stretching from Wyoming to Indiana.

I had held the gig since 2017. It extended a three-decade
string of Kafkaesque jobs. For puny wages I'd filed billion-dollar
profit results in annual corporate reports kept in a silent library
above the boisterous New York Stock Exchange floor, proofread
patent applications for a law firm (including a plan to convert
a pancake freezing apparatus into a producer of frozen umbili-
cal cord stem cells), administered the lost and found box (goggles,
swim caps) at an aquatic center, vetted voluminous issues of the
Facts On File *World News Digest*, weighed rugalach at a Brooklyn

3

bakery with dear teardrop string dispensers dangling from the ceiling, occupied a festooned cottage at Macy's flagship store on Herald Square, where as Santa I received—and sorted—dream information.

The eICU nurses and intensivists had their mission to save lives. I had a need to eat plus a respect for weird jobs because each position brought me into regular contact with the routines and aspirations, pleasures and disappointments, of the workaday world. The intensity of common experience never failed to enrich, and challenge, my understanding of the America I wrote about.

On March 10, the day South Dakota reports its first COVID cases (including one death), I note the unit operates exactly as usual while the plasma TV on the wall features reports of the epidemic's dawn in Manhattan.

The next shift the same. And the shift after that.

An eICU employee in my position answers the phone and transfers calls, a traffic controller. Minds the virtual census list. Does rudimentary charting on patients—temperature, Glasgow Coma Score, fluid intake/output. Listens to the complaints and exhaustion of clinicians who call, and fulfills requests of RNs seated at desks near the secretarial station. The eICU nurses and I are based in Sioux Falls, an urban area of roughly 250,000 (including suburbs) in the county of Minnehaha in eastern South Dakota. In 2015 Anne, a poet, and I moved here from Harlem. We each had old Midwest roots that needed further unearthing. We wildly hoped to live cheaper—reduce day-job stress—write more.

The first people to inhabit the area are thought to have arrived about 10,000 years ago. The Lakota named the spot Watpaipakshan (trans. where the Sioux River bends). Over 140 languages are spoken in Sioux Falls. More Lost Boys—former child soldiers in the Sudanese Civil War—are settled here than anywhere else in the nation. Digital billboards broadcast public health messages in Amharic and Swahili and Arabic. The Iowa state line and the Minnesota state line are less than twenty miles away. The eICU staff reports to a nondescript one-story building near I-90 with flags planted around it—often at half-mast, given the recent preponderance of mass shootings. The building looks like a strip mall without stores where there should be stores. The eICU doctors—linked to the unit via phone and camera— are based around America and the world (Michigan to India) because of the scarcity of specialists in ICU care. Telehealth nurses often are drawn from a pool of local professionals who can no longer handle the physicality of bedside care but have decades of valuable experience to offer.

A support specialist sees the patient into the system and sees them out—discharging a name, a lifetime, to HOME or FLOOR or DEATH. Admitting a patient into the virtual census involves typing data into a program called eCare Manager: name, account number, admitting doctor, diagnosis. From then on data from a bedside monitor (pulse rate, for example) flow continuously into an in-house patient file that is separate from the patient's official electronic medical record (EMR). The in-house file captures only data generated while the patient is being cared for by the eICU unit. For historicity the EMR is consulted. Each EMR has its own rhythm of connection to memorize and not get panicked by. Most require a username and password to be entered twice. Essentially the patient treated in the telehealth setting is a collation of all these programs and their lab numbers, MRI images, notes. That plus the face on a screen delivered by a Philips camera and the room racket of voices, machines.

The gospel prior to the pandemic was that eICU nurses and doctors *never* replace bedside providers, and instead offer the support of a second eye, a second opinion, the force of collaboration to ensure, when all works smoothly, better care. But what health care entity could possibly operate smoothy when pressured by unprecedented circumstances?

The eICU—created in 2004 by this hospital system to aid its own small (twenty-five beds or fewer) rural hospitals with critical patients—faced an immediate problem after the virus arrived. Two difficulties, actually.

In this two-week period after the first local infection was reported by KELO I heard that many staff members—especially the South Dakota natives—just couldn't believe that a scourge devastating the East Coast would eventually worm its way into the nursing homes, factories, tribal lands, day care centers, schools, prisons of the Upper Midwest. In the break room RNs assured each other: "Well, maybe it won't hit us hard out here. We're South Dakota." Translation: *What happens on the East Coast never has anything to do with us.* I often gently reminded coworkers of my connections with family and friends in New York City in an attempt to erode the wall of this assumption, with mixed results.

The second problem, though, was much larger: how to quickly, sensibly, scale up an intricate patchwork of unit and off-site hardware to triple or even quadruple the number of patients served. As many unit employees struggled to believe in the approaching disaster, very convinced upper level administrators were scrambling to develop a frontline response to the virus crossing state lines—a strategy to present to eICU supervisors who would then present it to us who worked the floor.

What would that strategy look like? How would I be involved in a support role? Could I handle it? Should I? This wasn't my career, was it? Yet I had a duty too.

I had a sudden sense—as I stood at my post under the wall TV—that whatever did ensue response-wise and casualty-wise, there was an imperative to witness and record what happened to patients and my friends the nurses, especially since spending time around them had taught me that—though labeled health care heroes—they were often forced to function within hierarchies that encouraged obedience rather than dialogue.

I had rarely worked with a nurse who felt her workplace concerns had been listened to well enough, and taken seriously enough, by those "above," mostly men. One of the most experienced nurses had lived through a time when it was not unheard of for a doctor to strike a nurse he was unhappy with for some reason. And each female doctor I had worked with had her own old and new stories of being insulted and ignored by colleagues of the opposite sex. Telehealth did not defuse the dynamic but offered it a new setting.

I decided I must take field notes of the developing event to capture the real-time reality of the telehealth response to the crisis in rural areas and the small cities of the paved plains. It would also be my best chance of engaging the circumstances personally, and making it through. Images and stories pinned for good to pages, not part of the on-screen flow of seen, erased, seen, erased. Pictures of resourceful coworkers facing resource shortfalls, pictures of technology colliding with calamity.

The eICU relied not only on hardware and software but also on expert advice of IT support personnel. The names of the best of these staff members had a divine resonance to us who were lost without them. *Casey. Brett. Michael.* What would happen if the census grew, and with it the IT problems, but not the IT staff? What if the IT staff got sick? Telehealth had this aura of abracadabra, but it was wires, man. Typed codes and plugs—lenses that got smudged and needed to be wiped clean—this team of people and machines. And as humans could falter so could cameras and microphones, and each tech failure had to be addressed at the same time as patients were being treated.

Of course nobody knew what was going to occur. We prayed, each of us, in our own way, for outcomes better than the worst possible outcomes. Then what happened happened. What I, at least, never figured on.

March 25
Birth of the Three-Armed Nurse

7:00 a.m. Lockdown protocol in effect at eICU building for safety purposes: no visitors, only the SW entrance is open. On entering, each employee is subjected to a temperature check and is asked, "Have a cough?" Arrive worried about friends and loved ones in New York City: fifteen hundred plus cases there now. Arrive with an inch-long burn blister on middle finger of right hand from brushing handle of a cast-iron pan last night when checking on roasting parsnips. Arrive forty-five minutes late because the automatic garage door refused to lift, leaving the car marooned inside. Double lockdown. I had to ask my supervisor to come pick me up, as no taxi services answered my calls. I waited for her on the front steps of our home, dressed in hunter-green scrubs. All eICU employees are required to wear scrubs to enhance the ambiance of care. A fact twisted around and around in my mind as I waited: 152 ICU beds in South Dakota—the governor, Kristi Noem (R), has announced that 300,000 cases are to be expected eventually.

8:00 a.m. Unit consists of eight stations crammed into a sporadically ventilated, windowless tan room that has at one end what we call "the glass bowl"—an enclosed bridge—where visitors are taken to view what an eICU is. (Trump administration officials have stood there. Eli Saslow, reporter from the *Washington Post*, stood there.) Each station is enveloped by wings of three large computer screens. On the screens the figures of patients sometimes flicker as if they were made of fire. Images of suffering have a mirage-like quality that the sounds of screams do not. Desks rise and fall at the push of a button. Four of the stations are unoccupied today. On one wall is a wide screen that allows the two nurses and me to see coworker Dr. S in Michigan, near Detroit.

9:00 a.m. I pick up the phone, I say my assigned lines in the drama: "eICU, Support Specialist Ben. How can I help you?" Phone rings again: repeat. The unit is an echo of a real ICU, but the removal from bedside also intensifies the importance of providing callers with a crisp, calming, productive human connection. The will to care has to be there. It cannot be allowed to flag. The words stay the same, infused by fresh energy.

After I admit a patient into the census system, the nurse or the doctor can click on the camera icon next to the name to get visual access to the room—its blankets, its tubes, its trouble—in Missouri or Minnesota or Iowa or Nebraska or North Dakota.

10:00 a.m. Because I believe in the power of rituals, and because it helps deal with the stress of the job, during my shifts I always ask at 3:00 p.m.: "Does anyone want tea?" Then repair to my locker to access my stash and fill any requests. At this early hour, however, for the first time, I am asked: "What about some tea?" Any excuse to step away, to rest eyes, stretch legs, I jump on. Green tea for Nurse H. Wild sweet orange for Nurse W.

Our hospital organization happens to be a religiously affiliated nonprofit operation. Both nurses express anger over the actions of another nonprofit hospital in the area with a different religious affiliation. That institution has not only not stopped doing elective procedures, they have increased the volume of elective procedures in order to conduct as many surgeries as possible before COVID patients disrupt the money stream. "Over eighty on Monday!" Nurse W notes how this squanders personal protective equipment (PPE) and crucial drugs like propofol that have to be administered to vented patients.

11:00 a.m. Nurse H worries about "all of the ventilators" going to New York City, leaving none for the rest of the nation.

She explains that as a middle child she always got the raggy hand-me-downs from her older sister—it makes her dread coming in second in situations.

12:00 p.m. Dr. S tells one of our nurses: "If you are [a COVID patient] placed on a vent your chances of recovery are cut in half." More bad news: there is one positive COVID case on a floor at the South Dakota minimum-security women's prison, and eight inmates from that floor have escaped. Then an Indiana nurse calls, tells of a man there who contracted the virus during a Sunday church service and was dead within the week.

2:00 p.m. Bold sign on a restroom door commands WASH HANDS. It would be nice if truly hot water gushed from taps in there, but it never has. The reality is that more and more WASH HANDS signs are posted around the facility as the ability to WASH HANDS continues to be hindered by the lack of hot water. I scrub longer as if this will make up for LWS: lukewarm water situation. I scrub in a new way due to the Band-Aid over the burn blister. I pump foamy soap into unharmed hand, then scrub that hand lightly, front and back, with just the unbandaged tips of my harmed hand. It is as if I am playing runs on a mini piano at the end of my wrists. I imagine receiving a patent for the process, donning a tux, giving hand-washing demos as a recording of Debussy plays in the background. Reveries like this make it more joyful to work for less than fifteen dollars an hour when you have an MA in English.

I receive word from Anne that our garage door has been fixed, and share the news. A twelve-hour shift is like being on a long car trip: no secrets. My tale prompts stories from the nurses about how when they were teens wanting to have a ripsnorting good time they drove around aiming their garage-door openers at random garages of strangers, speeding away if the doors lifted.

3:00 p.m. I walk around the parking lot where I watch for doves and sparrows and hawks and the bird called the killdeer.

I have an index card and a pen in the pocket of my coat in case I get an idea. Many short stories have started on a break, as my mind approached interesting ICU issues of human fragility and resiliency from angles natural to me. During one walk I had the sudden image of a dead patient being lifted and the lifters seeing, on the bed, a large bluish egg that immediately complicated things. Was the man actually dead? Or living on in a new form? His wife: what did she feel? Today no epiphanies. Today I notice a bumper sticker on an SUV back window that maybe was funny once but not now: THE EMPIRE DOES NOT CARE ABOUT YOUR STICK FIGURE FAMILY.

5:00 p.m. Upset doctor from Site 6 calls. Indicates he has a "COVID-19 probable" but that there is no negative-pressure room [safer for clinicians] at his tiny hospital. I transfer the worry to Dr. S. Nurse H remarks: "No negative-pressure room? I thought they all had to have at least one negative-pressure room!" Turns out there is one such room at the site, but it is not outfitted with our technology. Can an adjustment be made?

There used to be only two ways an eICU doctor or nurse could "camera" into a room: (1) camera mounted on ceiling; (2) camera on a portable cart. Because of the potential increase in patient volume, eICU iPads have begun to be distributed far and wide to hospitals—including this one—to offer yet a third possibility of connection. Only no one in the unit with me today has tried this option. Nurse W tells me she will try if the cart option fails. I thank her. I now have a thing to tell the Site 6 nurse who will be upset if the cart option fails. It's a job of thinking ahead.

6:00 p.m. At Site 10 there is a "crasher"—as nurses call it—code situation. Codes are generally run by site staff, with our doctor observing, available to advise if necessary. And, during this hour, another crasher at Site 11. Nurse H and Dr. S deal with those fraught situations as Nurse W and I try to address the technology riddle at Site 6.

Nurse at Site 6 calls. The mobile camera cart is finally in the room with the patient in need of our assistance: "Can you see him?" I click camera icon. Error message. I ask if the patient's account number had been accurately entered into the cart—which must be done for it to function. She thinks it has been, but. . . . Ordinarily I would quickly read the number off to her and request she enter the figures as soon as she can, but now I pause. Think: "How can I ask her to go into the room with a COVID-probable patient to fix an account number when I can't be sure she has the appropriate protective gear on?" I say: "We need to get the number into the cart—but don't go in there if you can't do it safely." She puts another nurse on the phone without answering. This nurse informs me that she has worked at the hospital for ten years and never entered a number into any cart whatsoever. I decide to put our IT staff in touch with these nurses and do. It is determined the cart is not working because the outlet in the negative-pressure room will not function with the mobile cart plug.

The next thing is to try the iPad ploy. Nurse W locates iPad instructions in an email. She follows the steps and manages to contact the patient, question him about his medical history. Then our doctor is able to view and assess the patient—to a point. The big difficulty? Not the connection. It's that the iPad must be cradled by the nurse in the room wearing protective gear. She must change the angle as instructed by the doctor, which is not easy. It leaves her with one hand free to do the many other things for the patient that must be done. "A dinosaur process," gripes Nurse W when the interaction concludes. She turns completely away from screens to tell me this.

What will happen—we both wonder—when there are twenty or thirty iPad scenarios playing out at the same time? Yet scarier still is not offering hospitals that have requested more coverage any option. And, I think, if you look at it another way, a one-armed nurse backed up by our nurse, is, well, a three-armed nurse in total.

March 26–27
Call of the Killdeer

7:00 p.m. Nice light on the drive in: sharp shadows of ash trees and telephone poles cutting across the Minnesota Avenue pavement. Unusual image of a possum waddling on one side of a fence near the airport, small, frustrated barking dogs on the other side. I prepare for shifts by listening to jazz. Tonight: looping clarinet lines of Artie Shaw because his is the nearest CD within reach in the front seat. The big-band leader's theme song is blaring as I arrive in the eICU parking lot. It is entitled "Nightmare."

One after the other I open the ten programs needed to do my job of list minding, data charting. I tag phone-bank buttons with the names of nurses and doctors I'll be working with for the next twelve hours. I cut strips out of sticky notes to make the tags, print names, stick strips next to buttons. The job feels in control once the buttons are tagged. I can handle anything then! Ten calls in ten minutes. Two calls a minute. A surprising amount of paper flies around an eICU. The nurses in the unit work off a paper census like I do. Tag phones like I do. The phones look as if they could use a shave.

8:00 p.m. At Site 27 there are designated "dirty nurses" and "clean nurses." The "dirty" work with the COVID patients. The "clean" with the other patients. An upset "dirty nurse" calls to complain about her plight. She says, "I have no children. But I have relatives with preexisting conditions. Is it fair I have to take a chance on infecting them?"

9:00 p.m. Dr. M in India calls to complain that he cannot access the EMR associated with Site 19. I connect him to IT help based in North Dakota.

10:00 p.m. There is a phrase in eICU lingo for being put on a vent. The nurses will say, "He bought himself a vent," or "She bought herself a vent." The nurses have already designated a subcategory of virus patients: "Another nursing-home COVID person."

I think of my in-laws in Brooklyn, both eighty years old, now locked down. They've been only kind to me. They both attended the University of Minnesota, ending up in New York City in 1964 when Jim was hired by a Manhattan law firm. We share a love of music, conversation, and good food. Gail has taught me more about cooking than anyone else. I grew up eating frozen TV dinners—on the good nights. She made sure her two daughters had fresh food. Tonight they have ordered carryout from Queen Restaurant—the place with the short maître d' with a sandpaper voice. Anne sends me the photo of the entrees they chose: veal marsala, veal piccata. I think of Tolan, our friend at New York–Presbyterian Hospital, the biomed tech. I think of our other friend, Leigh, an administrator at the Brooklyn Hospital Center. What must they be enduring at this hour? I listen to New York City updates on 1010 WINS. When I can't absorb more updates I listen to Sheila Anderson's late-night jazz show on WBGO. "I'm with you," she says in a perfect radio voice, a little scratchy, always sounding on the edge of emotion, keeping it real, but never flipping into turbulence. "Keep your ears here," she says. She lives in Harlem near where we used to live. Duke Ellington called it Sugar Hill.

11:00 p.m. I admit a probable COVID patient to Site 8 and discover the mobile-cart camera in the room does not work. I call the site, ask, "Is the cart plugged in?" Nurse plugs cart in. I test camera again. It works now. The room is crowded with young nurses wearing full-body protective gear or "pappers." To me they resemble beekeeper outfits.

I remind myself to remember always to ask nurses at certain sites the "plugged in" question. The smallest of the thirty-four sites, in ordinary times, don't have many eICU patients—sometimes only one a month, if that many. But I can forget which sites these are.

The hodgepodge of different types (different eras) of technology reflects how the eICU has evolved since it was inaugurated over sixteen years ago—grown via accretion, new procedures instituted as new sites are taken on, while the older sites often are allowed to continue using antiquated devices and protocols the nurses and doctors are familiar with. The crisis may make the lack of uniformity more glaring.

12:00 a.m. Besides the N95 mask shortage—which exists at some of our sites even though none have felt the brunt of the pandemic yet—there is also at one hospital a perplexing shortage of artificial tears. Dr. M orders an "ointment" to be used instead. Little details like this have a way of attaching to the imagination. *The supply of fake tears drying up as too many genuine reasons to cry appear around every single American.*

1:00 a.m. There exist ten COVID-positive patients at Site 30, but the eICU unit has been directed by the bedside staff to "follow" only one. How can that be the case? I consult orders for the ten: indeed, we've been asked only to help out with one. Is it a money-saving measure—given that here our service is billed by the number of patients served? "Telehealth" has a universal ring . . . but every now and then, since I started working in the unit, I have listened to various nurses examine the ethics of utilization: "What if these families knew *their loved one* was not getting the support *another patient* received? Would they be happy about that? I don't think so. I really don't."

3:00 a.m. On a three-lap walk around a dark parking lot I hear high-pitched fifing of the killdeer. The lot is bookended by Pepsi distributorship warehouses to the south, and the headquarters of POET, an ethanol producer, to the north. Killdeer effusions span the entire distance. These birds prefer scurrying across pavement to flying. They look like New Yorkers used to look during rush hour in Grand Central.

When I reenter the building at the designated door I encounter a young man in jeans and young woman in jeans standing at the table where temp screening is done. They are the cleaning help. No one sits there to take temps at this hour. The young man draws a finger across his forehead, mimicking the path of the temp-taking device. He does not know much English. It's almost as if he is making the sign of the cross in the dim hallway. I nod, meaning: "I'll help." I call an eER doctor. He does the screening. (The twenty-four-hour eER unit—or virtual emergency room—is also located off "the glass bowl.")

4:00 a.m. More confusion at Site 27. There's a COVID-positive patient there on BiPAP, a type of less invasive ventilation. The BiPAP causes the virus to aerosolize, or enter the air. The "dirty" nurse treating the patient does not have a complete protective outfit—she only has a mask. "Can I enter the room?" she asks our Nurse F. "What's your hospital policy?" Nurse F responds. "No idea," says the site nurse. Soon the patient is intubated, which resolves the problem. The vent is a sealed system . . . unless a cap pops off. Nurse R theorizes this particular patient may have been vented to solve the PPE quandary instead of for medical reasons. Nurses are suspicious. They have reasons to suspect. Nurses are also pragmatic. Other nights I have heard accounts of violent meth ODs being vented to protect staff. The vent as a lifesaver for those standing *next to* its drone.

5:00 a.m. Tea time to keep the spirits up. I set out the baby-blue pot of hot water, the china cups, the six tea options. Nurse F chooses Green Dandelion. Nurse R, Sleepytime. I have a V8. Patients are rousing around the Midwest. Calls for sedation orders.

7:00 a.m. I walk across the lot to my car. Vivid orange cracks of light in the dawn sky. When I turn the key in the ignition, I hear trumpets. The rest of "Nightmare" is playing.

March 30
The Egg Bake in the Storm's Eye

7:00 a.m. On the ten-minute drive to work, I pass, as usual, the cathedral, the state penitentiary, and Joe Foss Field, the local name for the airport. Each structure pertinent to the crisis that calls for spiritual wherewithal, inflicts imprisonment, and complicates travel. A New Yorker is now dying every six minutes of the COVID virus.

10:00 a.m. "Want an egg bake?" I turn. A nurse from the eER stands a few feet behind me, clutching a tray of aluminum take-out containers sealed with white lids. "A caterer sent these for the doctors and there are extra." "What's an egg bake?" I ask, not wanting to know. "Eggs with stuff in them. Different stuff. All sorts of stuff." It sounds like high-calorie goo. I don't need any goo. I point to my pear. She retreats. There is a policy I follow for my own health: *Do not eat the free food at work.*

12:00 p.m. I admit the first patient five hours into the shift. Not a COVID patient. Seventeen of the twenty-four ICU beds at the largest hospital we support are empty. News coverage oozes across the TV screen next to the other wall screen some call "the doc in the box" because it displays one of the off-site intensivists on shift poised in front of their screens. New York governor Andrew Cuomo issues a plea for health care workers to come to help New Yorkers. Images of bodies being loaded into refrigerated trucks outside hospitals—the surreal field hospital erected in Central Park. "We're in the eye of the storm," says Nurse W, softly. There are a few COVID-infected holdovers from yesterday on our census. These are in the easternmost states we provide service to.

2:00 p.m. Nurse W recounts seeing three party buses in front of a local bar called the 18th Amendment last Friday. She shakes her head again. There is no shelter-in-place order in South Dakota. Paul TenHaken (R), the mayor of Sioux Falls—the state's biggest city—has his thinking cap on, trying to decide the proper course of action. Both he and the governor quite often use the word "data." Following "data." Waiting on "data." COVID could kill 4 percent of those who get it—that's what I read. And the state's leader has announced that 30 percent of residents—or 300,000—could be infected, meaning 3,600 deaths. What is there to wait for? To follow? Other than stringent safety measures?

4:00 p.m. Things get busier: four admits in an hour, none COVID. One thousand confirmed infections in North Dakota, but the two ICU beds we watch there are unused.

6:00 p.m. Nurse E again communicates her feeling this place won't be hit hard because it is not densely populated. Nurse W counters: "But it only takes one to spread it everywhere."

My gaze keeps darting among the various screen glows, various screen scripts. One person has to be a multiplicity of seers when it comes to the many screens that define telehealth. At times I am a seeker looking through a screen trying to see other people and places. At times I am a robot who just looks at a screen, charting patient lab results. 10,000 DEAD IN UNITED STATES IN FIVE WEEKS, CNN reports. The screen nearest to my face represents the tiniest sliver of that data, but it, and the TV screen above, are two pictures slowly being spliced together each shift to create one arc—one history—one fever conjoined.

March 31
The River Lethe Machine

8:00 a.m. An Indiana nurse who alternates between bedside and telehealth reports that in the ICU at the main hospital in her area there are thirty-six beds and all but six are occupied by vented COVID patients. An hour away, at another hospital, eighty-six workers have tested positive for the virus. She has been instructed to use the same mask for a week.

10:00 a.m. Since I started working in the unit in 2017, directly to the right of my desk has been a copy machine that attracts traffic. Now, directly to the left of the desk is this new contraption. It will stay, I am told. It consists of a dangling headset plus a wide screen on a rod suspended over a little desk where a keyboard rests. Attached to the top of the rod like the eye of a fly is an oval camera. It is there, I am told, because the eICU has been informed that when a COVID patient goes into cardiac arrest the code will not be run by bedside staff but by our doctor in Michigan or India or Israel and a nurse standing at this device, serving as "recorder," calling out pulse rates at regular intervals. The strategy is designed to protect as many local practitioners as possible from getting infected during a surge. Eyes roll in the unit as the news spreads. "Let's hope there will not be any," someone mutters, more magical thinking, but her face tells the truth that she is quite worried. Telehealth is still a fairly young concept, growing in fits and starts as young ideas do, a confusing as well as a hope-inducing force. This gawky machine is the surest official sign so far that we are all in new, threatening territory. The first test happens as I try to go on answering the phone: "eICU, Support. . . ." "Testing. Owatonna, are you there? . . . are you there? Owatonna?" Instant concerns arise regarding the quality of the audio feed because some human beings do need to be in the room with the patient— an RN pushing meds and a respiratory therapist, plus the person doing the CPR. They can't clearly hear directions from our doctor when draped with gear. I think of one name for this device rigged to channel a current of dying Midwesterners: the River Lethe Machine (RLM). In Greek *lethe* means oblivion.

11:00 a.m. Take one quick parking-lot lap to escape the chill technological sight of the machine with the official Orwellian name of PolyCom RealPresence cart. Cooing doves pair off amid greening perimeter shrubs. Spring is trying to arrive. A pothole filled with water glimmers like an inkwell awaiting a six-foot-tall pen. When the killdeer rises, its fanning tail reveals apricot feathers framed in white.

12:00 p.m. My friend at New York–Presbyterian reports that they are doubling up on ICU beds.

2:00 p.m. Nurse G admits: "I worry that in this time I'm thinking too much about myself and my situation and not enough about others." As hard as nurses can be on one another, they are usually hardest on themselves. I nod. Fear increases self-centeredness.

3:00 p.m. Is a patient in a room at Site 19 gone? The name has fallen off the EMR roster. I just called the site about another matter and the nurse sounded harried. Another call will make her bad day worse. I must take a peek into the room myself. I don't like to do this. Each shift I use the camera as few times as possible. I am allowed to use it—some of the other support specialists use cameras as a major tool in the effort to maintain an accurate census—but I have never felt comfortable with it because if I was in a sad state in a bed, struggling to breathe, I'd not want a member of the Kafka Corps of List Minders looking in for the sole purpose of making sure the paperwork was absolutely correct. But in a case like this I must. When I click the camera icon I hear the real item hum. First things seen are the mottled ceiling tiles. Then the lens dips and swings, and the bed comes into view, empty, dirty sheets bunched, waiting for removal by the room prepper. When I click DISCONNECT the room far away in Missouri—every color in it a nauseating variation of tan—vanishes and bold blue letters appear on a pure white background: PHILIPS, the camera maker's name.

4:00 p.m. This is one of those times during the shift when I manually enter urine output data into eCare Manager for patients being treated at the few sites that are still equipped (or ill-equipped) with technology so primitive that not a byte of data flows from room machines into our file. If there is no output I type: "No opu." There is obvious poetry to the phrase. As all codes go through the RLM, all pee goes through me.

7:00 p.m. On the way home—before passing the airport, the prison, the spires of St. Joseph, the Good Samaritan nursing home—I roll by a bait shop. The marquee out front reads FISHING IS SOCIAL DISTANCING. As has been the case for the last four evenings, when I reach the driveway I smell lumber burning in neighbor David's large pit. It is his curious way of dealing.

April 1
The Yellow Glove

7:00 a.m. The facts we pick up on during the onslaught of facts—those that don't stick, those that do—are how we reconstitute reality under the disassembling pressure of the pandemic. Gas $1.44 a gallon. "Cupboards bare at the Strategic Stockpile." The Empire State Building bathed in red and white light. The yellow glove I had yesterday and somehow lost on the walk to the car after the shift or the walk from the driveway into the house or somewhere else along the way. This a focal point for emotion as I enter the building. Like a nine-year-old, I want to cry.

8:00 a.m. I see the latest edition of the iPad distribution list. A spreadsheet pages long.

9:00 a.m. I have another friend in New York City who is still going to work, but he does not work at a hospital. Ivan is a guard at the PNC Bank across from Madison Square Garden. It is slow in there. He has plenty of time to be on his phone. Throughout each shift he sends me links to inspiring musical performances on YouTube. He's cheering me on, and his is the city in hideous crisis. That emotional largesse seems to characterize a certain kind of New Yorker. Billy Eckstine singing "Somewhere Over the Rainbow." O. C. Smith's "Little Green Apples." "Come Softly to Me," the Fleetwoods. Short messages sometimes accompany the links: *The music keeps my heart beating! Love you Ben!*

10:00 a.m. Latest misbegotten corporate attempt to boost morale: a bag of free green and white (company colors) sunglasses in the break room for the taking. But there are no windows in the eICU. But it is the light we need the most.

11:00 a.m. Dr. S sends the shift crew a copy of an article on the virus. The author is Paul G. Auwaerter, professor of medicine at Johns Hopkins University. One sentence sticks: "Origin is uncertain although bats implicated."

12:00 p.m. The treatment technique of proning, flipping a patient onto their stomach to increase oxygen flow to the lungs, is being used on COVID patients to delay, and maybe even eliminate, the need for intubation. Nurses note the aggressiveness of the tactic is warranted by the frightening fact that a COVID patient can go from breathing normally to intubated in eight hours or less. I am instructed to identify COVID patients specifically on in-house census lists like I identify TRAUMA patients and TRANSPLANT patients.

1:00 p.m. Raking through an EMR Nurse U discovers that one of our patients with pneumonia has not received antibiotics for twenty-four hours. "People are forgetting the basics," she snaps, picks up the phone, informs our doctor, and the medicine gets into the man.

2:00 p.m. Another mock code using the River Lethe Machine is attempted. Nurses in Minnesota can't hear the voice of our doctor in Michigan even when she shouts.

3:00 p.m. The Benedictine sisters in Yankton, South Dakota, ring their monastery bells shortly after 3:00 p.m. each day, a call for prayer during the crisis.

While walking parking-lot laps under wires strung with doves, I pull out my phone and call an artistic collaborator in Brooklyn to cheer him on. Dale picks up. He is outside—first time in a week. Waiting in line to get into the Park Slope Co-op. He expresses a deep feeling of disconnection with things in the city like the field hospital in Central Park. He sees the crisis playing out on a screen just like me, 1,361 miles away.

7:00 p.m. Each time my temperature is checked a colored dot is applied to my badge. I have four of them. Today's is yellow like my lost glove. I see it again when I swipe out.

April 6
Miracle Acres

7:00 a.m. On April 3 the governor warned residents that as many as 600,000 people could be infected by the virus—double the previous projection. She continues to balk at issuing a statewide shelter-in-place order. What she has done is declare April 8 a Statewide Day of Prayer. I keep wondering how leaders of the state's two largest hospital systems—including the one I work for—can stand on the same press-conference stage and not raise their voices in protest. I wonder how they sleep.

Heightened sensitivity to the fragility of life lends one new eyes. Today, when commuting to work, just past the airport, ahead on the pavement, I spot a run-over creature, white and fluffy, and hit the brakes as if that could help.

8:00 a.m. I learn the term *Crisis Support Model*. It is the name for service that rural hospitals desperate for telehealth support are being offered at the last moment. CSM consists of the iPads and the River Lethe Machine. I am haunted by the notion that if its dark screen does eventually brighten, death coursing across it, the losses will essentially go unmarked due to the volume. When one of my supervisors looks at the dark screen he thinks this out loud: "It's just going to be a nightmare, no matter how you look at it. I tried to tell them—it'll be a shit show." Should I do a drawing each time I hear someone die? Write a word? I'm not a clinician. Art somehow has to answer.

10:00 a.m. Tests of iPad protocol continue. "Would earbuds help? Wireless earpiece?" It might, a tester indicates. On the spot a decision is made to get some and try that way of delivering audio to frontline nurses behind face shields.

12:00 p.m. Admit first COVID patient of the day—currently all but one of our positive patients are at this single site in south-eastern Indiana.

1:00 p.m. THREE LIONS WITH DRY COUGHS AT BRONX ZOO! TV headline proclaims. The dry cough of a lion. Another thing to try to imagine because it exists.

2:00 p.m. Dr. D hasn't worked a shift for weeks. When that happens I get urgent calls from him about expired passwords and related cyber difficulties. For help unraveling the gnarl I call an eICU employee working from home. She tells me her four stir-crazy kids are in the backyard next to a cornfield they can run into, extending their play by acres, miracle acres, at a time of shrinking space for almost everyone else.

April 7
Shadow of the First Crocus

7:00 a.m. On the commute I note a peach-striped, yellow orb in the sky over the vacant airport parking lot: it looks like a sun become a moon. Yesterday, a purple crocus bloomed in our backyard. In past years the event has been powerful medicine, making Anne and me feel better, a definitive finger pointing away from ice and mud and toward the lushness of spring leaves and petals. This year it is not at all clear what is being pointed at. Four masks have arrived in the mail. Anne's mother sewed them in Brooklyn on the same cabinet-model Sear's machine she used to make Anne's wedding dress and the vest (made out of dark green material left over from the wedding dress) I wore with my vintage light green wedding jacket, and the pink curtains for the French doors of our apartment in Harlem, and the dragonfly-pattern covering for the cushions that fit into the window seat there.

8:00 a.m. Another potential difficulty arises with the Crisis Support Model. Only one person at a time can view the patient via the iPad—either our nurse or our doctor or a member of the site staff trying to avoid entering the room for safety reasons. Choreographing quick trade-offs under pressure could be hard. And they must be quick.

9:00 a.m. Nurse E: "It scares me when the nurses at our hospitals have no fear. One [measure] up or one down on a drip—that can cause a patient to die." Nurse H: "Tell you this, if I had a relative in the ICU I'd camp out there, never leave."

But what does advocating for a relative's good care look like if you are not allowed to step into the hospital lobby? Can't see what is going on? Should there be a teleadvocacy option for relatives, an instant way for them to corner the attention of a doctor in the same way they can fly to the side of a loved one via FaceTime? How many lives will be lost during the duration of the pandemic because a patient has no family member or friend in the room to advocate for them—to concentrate only on their outcome?

Nurses I have worked with over the past two years have also often hit that alarming note about never wanting to leave a loved one alone in an ICU or in any hospital ward: they have seen many mistakes happen. Many needless deaths. That is, many sloppy, arrogant doctors protected by a fraternity of silence and many mediocre nurses tolerated because they will work holidays and nights for you. Doctors who "perfed" colons while doing colonoscopies. Doctors who refused to coordinate patient care with other doctors, leading to harm from drug mismatches. Nurses who at the start of each shift flooded their patients with sedatives to keep them quiet. Nurses who could not "hang a bag" or "run a line." There was one of these nurses hiding out in the open in the eICU; I had seen her turn her back on EKG rhythms on her screens to spend twenty minutes criticizing the poor performance of a Target employee that had not carried her items to her car fast enough. Another day, after failing a CPR test on an automated dummy six times, this nurse let other nurses take the test for her. They offered, desperate to get her to stop talking about failing the test six times. They had work to do! The dummy was wheeled into the unit. It had no legs: a torso on a table between my desk and the other stations across the aisle.

11:00 a.m. Nurse H calls a site and says as gently as is possible: "I'm worried about the man in 133. A little tachy [high heart rate]. He doesn't look good in the room. Or on paper. Has your doctor rounded yet? Yes? He didn't say too much, huh? He did see that his diastolic is elevated above 100? Well . . . if he saw it . . . we are out of the middle of it. Okay. I'll probably talk to you a little later."

12:00 p.m. Listening again to the twenty-four-hour Billie Holiday birthday broadcast on WKCR. Her blues speak to all blues. At the end of "Strange Fruit," Abel Meeropol's ferocious ballad about lynchings that she made famous, Holiday draws out the first syllable of "bitter" before the consonants bite down on the flow of air, cutting off the air. Death. Defeat. Resilience. For a singer she did not have a wide octaval range. Her talent was the reach of feeling, structure, knowledge.

3:00 p.m. Overhear the COVID hotline supervisor asking the receptionist at the front desk for more computers, more phones.

4:00 p.m. Report that a Walmart pharmacist in South Dakota has tested positive for COVID.

7:00 p.m. Thirty-two new cases in South Dakota today, the total now at 320. Two more deaths. In New York plans are in the works to convert St. John the Divine, a gigantic cathedral near Columbia University, into a hospital. If necessary, beds will be installed in the crypts.

April 9–10
It Got Cirino

7:00 p.m. In the new park in front of the new City Hall building stands a new statue of Martin Luther King Jr. The bronze is extending a hand of friendship to someone not there. On the commute I see this, and, too, in the distance the roof of the Smithfield pork-processing plant. Over eighty workers tested positive for the virus on Saturday. The cases represent one-fifth of the cases in the state—a total now up to 393 (23 percent increase since Tuesday). Anecdotal reports indicate that workers with temps over a hundred degrees have not just been allowed to keep working but encouraged to do so by a $500 "responsibility bonus" going to anyone who does not miss one April shift. The factory is still in operation this evening, a Thursday. In there are kill rooms where pigs die. In there are rooms that could mean death for workers who enter.

8:00 p.m. Dr. K is our coworker in Tel Aviv. She never demeans nurses, never belittles their suggestions. Most eICU nurses are not afraid of being challenged but want criticism to be constructive. Dr. K's voice is firm. She is renowned for her calm, her thorough notes, her decisiveness. Tonight a COVID patient at a site needs to be paralyzed in order that respiratory treatment can be safely delivered. "Have paralyzed," she writes. Any shift Dr. K works is a shift less touched by nonsense.

9:00 p.m. "How are your friends in New York?" I am asked. I relate that our first friend died yesterday. Early fifties. A psychotherapist. Wife. Two kids under the age of ten. The bad news came to us through a mutual friend in Brooklyn. We arranged to toast Cirino at the same time with nice Italian wine.

10:00 p.m. Phone rings. It's our telehealth nurse who also works bedside a few shifts a week. He is calling to let me know there is a new patient coming to his unit. Early seventies. Male. Smithfield plant worker. Situation grave. In a short time he has gone from needing three liters of oxygen per minute to fifteen liters. "Glassy" infiltrates on the lungs.

12:00 a.m. A bug afflicts the headset connected to Nurse H's tabletop phone. Audio is iffy. She jabs into a socket the cord of a headset from another station. Fixed. Then her keyboard AA batteries run down: she has to change out those. Stressful glitches, for at any moment she might hear an alarm sound, need to respond fast.

1:00 a.m. Today it's a hospital-gown shortage across America. According to officials, "protocols for the recycling of gowns are being crafted." The telehealth nurse working bedside tonight calls again for our support. He has a rich baritone voice. I worry about him in the live unit with the infected patients. He is less than two years from a lake-cabin retirement. There is an app on his phone that is continually counting down the time to liberation— counting the hours, the minutes, the seconds. He has shown it to me. He is one of many nurses potentially threatened not just by where they work but also by the environment of the hospital where a partner is employed. His wife is at the VA. Before nursing he was a truck dispatcher and then a pharmaceutical salesman. One nurse makes yogurt to wind down. Some nurses read long books. Some nurses hike at Good Earth State Park. He and his wife attend hockey games.

3:00 a.m. I pick up the phone and an Indiana nurse blurts, "I'm not positive"—the most positive thing she can think to say. I ask how she has been. She says she worked sixty hours last week. At the end of the marathon, she went home and slept for twelve hours, then got up and cut the lawn. "We have grass here," she says with tired wonder.

4:00 a.m. I hear the fifing call of the killdeers on my half-hour walk around the parking lot. There is not much wind. A semi angles out of the beverage distributorship, on the side a product name: LIFE WTR. An identical semi follows, both trucks I-90 bound.

5:00 a.m. I'm thinking about our friend that died. When a person is defined by movement, as Cirino was in my mind, it is all the more difficult to comprehend a sudden stilling. Helmeted, he raced up and down Manhattan avenues on his ten-speed. When he talked his arms often lifted and dropped like he was conducting an orchestra. His questions were epic in their brevity, their bluntness, their collective implications. I'll never forget the wild look in Cirino's eyes as he asked, "Ben, why do you write?" or "Ben, what is marriage?" It was like being in the clutches of the world's best, and perhaps most fearsome, interviewer. After these zingers he'd freeze and force me to answer by waiting until I mumbled some inadequate response to which he would respond with an "ahhhhh." The delicate wire rims and swaying big hair have been with me all night long, and will continue to be. He knew how to live. He was incredibly fun to be around. We had a mystical hobby of accidently bumping into each other in the largest city in America, he seeing me from a distance in the hive and swerving to a stop in the middle of Sixth or Seventh Avenue—risking an accident—to shout a greeting. The last time I ran into him was in Marcus Garvey Park, uptown. We had both been drawn to the same outdoor jazz concert starring pianists McCoy Tyner and Jason Moran. He had the good picnic supplies. Real napkins. Real fork and knife. The fine pinot grigio. Real wine glasses. He had taken the afternoon off from his practice. He had downed two-thirds of the bottle before we ran into each other. He gave me the rest, though it was so good it went down like a mere two tablespoons as he leveled me with queries about the life we were living on Convent Avenue with our writing. He showed me pictures of his wife, and their first child. He had an ambitious plan for the rest of the day: five stops before home.

6:00 a.m. Nurse H remarks: "I'm noticing these COVID patients, their ionized calcium is always low. I haven't seen that many yet. But it is a pattern."

7:00 a.m. The morning news scrolls across the wall TV as the shift nears its end. CAR MAKER IN INDIA HAS DESIGNED A CAR THAT LOOKS LIKE THE COVID VIRUS. . . . NBA LEGEND ABDUL-JABBAR DONATES 1,800 PAIRS OF GOGGLES USED AS PLAYER TO HEALTH CARE WORKERS. . . . QUEEN ELIZABETH'S DRESS-MAKER IS MAKING HOSPITAL GOWNS. . . . EASTER SERVICES TO BE HELD AT DRIVE-IN THEATERS IN THE SOUTH. . . . As I leave fresh staff arrives and temperatures are taken at the door. All week there have been complaints about the low-quality thermometers used for the screening. Readings are erratic. "They bought the cheapest ones," I've been told. Some nurses doing the checking have started bringing their thermometers from home.

April 13
Waving White Flags

7:00 a.m. Three hundred fifty cases of COVID can now be connected to the Smithfield plant. Friends from around the country are emailing me, concerned. "Keep safe" is the refrain.

More than five inches of snow fell yesterday, altering the commute landscape. The Good Samaritan nursing home is tucked under a sheet. While I am stopped at an intersection a swath of snow stuck on the windshield wiper of the car behind me catches my attention like a flag. Due to the infections at the Smithfield pork-processing plant, Sioux Falls now has more cases per capita than Chicago. On Saturday the governor and the mayor finally requested that the plant close. The next day, Easter, the ham holiday, the plant announced it would close indefinitely. This morning the CEO of Smithfield, Kenneth Sullivan, issued a statement warning that the nation's supply of meat is now endangered. The plant—controlled by the Hong Kong–based Shuanghui International Holdings Limited—supplies 5 percent of the pork sold in the United States or 130 million servings of pork per week. But the plant is not closed yet. It won't close until tomorrow, after remaining inventory is processed.

8:00 a.m. There are more than twice as many COVID cases on the census than any other morning I have worked since the crisis began. There are four Smithfield patients in the ICU at the big hospital we support in Sioux Falls, I'm told, and thirty others elsewhere in the facility. Nurses discuss ventilator-setting strategy. The main dilemma: "Turn the PEEP up on patients and risk trauma to the lungs? Turn the PEEP down and risk trauma to the brain?" ICU nurses, like soldiers, invent slang that gives them a feeling of control over chaos. They call the virus "Rona." They look at each other and smile and ask: "Are you there, Rona?" They look at me and ask that. "Are you there, Rona?" While I'm thinking: *What would you choose? Lung injury or brain injury?* It's like those questions my mentally ill mother would ask me as she walked me to school. "Honey, which limb would you choose to have amputated if you had to have one cut off?"

9:00 a.m. A nurse calls, relates she is having an awful time keeping her seventeen-year-old son at home. He is "all about making money." He works on machines at a firm not shut. He doesn't see what a big deal the whole thing is. She can't figure out how to help him conceive of the danger.

10:00 a.m. Governor Noem, flanked again by hospital executives, holds a presser announcing the state has been chosen as the site of the first large-scale trial of the controversial drug hydroxychloroquine. She adds: "Smithfield has done incredible work to put in infrastructure to protect their employees." But the plant isn't closed yet. No build-out of new structures can have begun. Earlier in the morning the mayor requested she declare a universal shelter-in-place order in the city. This is not addressed.

11:00 a.m. Am told by our Dr. S that a Sioux Falls intensivist expressed frustration to her about language barriers making it harder to treat the Smithfield patients.

12:00 p.m. A smiling supervisor stops by with a baggie full of masks sewn for our unit by volunteers. A number of the specimens resemble potholders with elastic straps. I pick the funny fellow of a mask made out of a tropical fabric sample. A fish where my mouth used to be, the blue of water, green of seaweed. The opposite of January cold in April, our weather today. But it does not fit. And because I tried it on, I am stuck with it as a backup to the homemade Brooklyn goods.

1:00 p.m. Almost all of the COVID patients in the ICU at the largest hospital in the city have been proned. It's a touchy procedure. Seven nurses were required to flip one of these patients earlier in the day. There are different methods. One involves using a blanket as a sling. I'm told patients can remain proned for seven hours. I'm told that after the procedure was done on one patient, oxygen saturation in the lungs jumped to 98 percent. Nurse O, clicking camera, shows me a proned patient, tubes leading from the body into the forest of bedside apparatus. The bed existing in a clearing. The noise of the camera like a woodland creature rustling around in leaves and needles.

2:00 p.m. Nurse O and Nurse G grew up in farming families, which is the case with many nurses I work with. Nurse O's father is a hog farmer. Nurse G's father runs feeder cattle. Neither dares to ask their parents about how business is, it's so bad.

Today in Tama, Iowa, a beef-processing plant also announced it was closing.

5:00 p.m. I've got my fucking parka on. I've got on a wool cap under the hood, mismatched gloves. Nothing will stop me from walking. Nothing ever has stopped me from walking, from childhood until now. I limped through the period of the torn meniscus when I was in my early fifties. As an obese ten-year-old I waddled like a penguin around my block, trying to get it together. Back then I never cried with tears. I grieved with dogged steps. Dunes of snow cover a large, empty lot near the parking lot I now walk around and around. The dunes like rows of proned pale figures. I've sometimes felt that there is a momentousness to every moment of existence waiting to be seen, caught, pried off the ritual and the dullness—but distraction and weariness intervene. The living, then, is mostly about continuing on.

6:00 p.m. On the wall in the break room is the new white board where coworkers try to write inspiring messages. One reads: "Keep looking up . . . God is in control." The continuing on takes this form of trust. Too, it takes the form of a neighbor boy carrying a plastic orange street pylon into his house. I saw that on Saturday. To put by his bed? In front of the stairs to his room? Divert evil! If you don't believe in God or pylons. . . .

7:00 p.m. Snowing again when I walk to the car in the parking lot, the snow mixed with light, the sun looking furry like lint. I steer down Fifty-Fourth Street, I turn onto Cliff Avenue, passing the Bar Code tavern. Seven trucks are parked in front—this is a scary amount given the rising rate of infection here. But for once there's not only horror at the sight but empathy, too. The pandemic has quieted the roar of America, sliced and flattened the roar into stray digital echoes—stretched thin moments of togetherness wrapping desolation. Are owners of the trucks dumb-stubborn? Or despairing to the point of destructiveness? Or believers in conspiracy theories that tell them there is actually no virus? Or seeking close company again to remind them why not to give up? Nearer to home I see a robin pecking reemerging greenness of turf.

April 14
Starting a Fire with Chicken Skin

7:00 a.m. Eighteen degrees. Driveway curds of ice crunching under tires. How a crisis reassembles even the most familiar landscape. The glassed-in portico of the Good Sam nursing home has come to look like an unprotected boxer's chin beside Minnesota Avenue. Stone syringes of the twin cathedral spires. The airport's air-control tower staffed with controllers that have few trajectories to guide. What happens between FedEx landings? Do they play poker? Smithfield finally shuttered. The penitentiary is the most static landscape element, hunkered behind curls of barbed wire.

8:00 a.m. I learn that two more COVID patients from Smithfield entered the ICU last night directly from the ER. Both vented, raising odds the cases will be fatal. Nurse E has something she thinks she needs to say to set the record straight: "It's their culture, you know. How they live—those workers—four to a small apartment." She nods in agreement with herself. Nurse G and I stare at her. I want to say: *It's the wage, you know, that dictates the size of the apartment you live in, and how you live there. . . .*

9:00 a.m. Admit to our census a COVID-positive patient from a South Dakota reservation. (So far there have been relatively few cases from the nine reservations in the state because of the wise decision of tribal leaders to stop outsiders from entering their territory.) This new case joins a prototypical mix of admits in a Midwest that before the pandemic faced an intertwined host of health crises. Into a bed we cover in Minnesota arrives a retired nurse who woke up with "Mexican jumping beans in her chest," as she describes atrial fibrillation. Into a bed we cover in Indiana arrives an LSD overdose found tripping at a gas station by police. Into a bed we cover in western Nebraska I admit another young patient who snorted too much fentanyl and was—as the nurses put it—"popped" back to life by two shots of Narcan. They all come from the ER, too.

10:00 a.m. No bedside data sets are flowing over into our eCare Manager system for a COVID patient in western Wyoming. For that to happen the patient has to be hooked up to the mobile cart there, and when I call to ask a nurse to do that, she explains that it is not safe to hook up the patient because the cart will get contaminated and not be able to serve one of the regular ICU patients that come in, OD or car crash or acute kidney injury (AKI) due to diabetes.

I wonder if millions of these carts should be manufactured by Sony like ventilators are now being made by Ford—this to prevent carts from being hoarded at resource-poor sites. Another question then occurs. Those iPads that have been sent to dozens of additional sites: how will they be adequately sanitized after being used?

11:00 a.m. Into a bed at a South Dakota site admit self-inflicted gunshot wound, sixteen years old.

Our doctor today in Michigan sends a message to the eICU group: "When is your governor going to do something?" The dark humor that gets ICU nurses through many hardships kicks in. One replies: "Haha! It's personal freedom! ☺"

Minutes before noon the first Smithfield COVID patient dies in a bed we monitor. I discharge the man to DEATH, sitting with the name a few minutes before tapping the digital button that will send all his data away too. I have done it many times before. This time, though, the act seems different. I'm too stunned to make a drawing—as I dreamed I might—to commemorate a life erased. Art cannot answer. I sit and stare at the letters of the name, the numbers of the birth date. On my commute I passed the one-hundred-year-old factory where he contracted the deadly virus. Close to home, this fatality, but no solidity of reality imbues the unit. The experience of the virtual cancels geography. The screens made the doctor in India feel closer to us than the Smithfield plant.

12:00 p.m. Any telehealth unit is prey to absurd interruptions by dialers of wrong numbers. I pick up, hear a grave, low, biblical voice demanding: "Connect me to Joseph." I hang up. Minutes later another ring. I pick up, hear the voice of a doctor in Montana requesting a psychological evaluation on a patient in a bed there. We don't do those.

2:00 p.m. The most successful test yet of the River Lethe Machine. The audio is almost too strong now. The unit fills with an eerie echo of a 1956 stadium PA system: *First down!*

3:00 p.m. On my break-time laps around the perimeter of the facility I spot a couple of killdeers scurrying across pavement, taking to the air, wings shuffling like cards: white, peach, gray. I blink. The afternoon is soaking in strong light that has followed the late snowstorm. Parking lot pebbles stand out to me. Pale smooth pebbles affixed with the sky's audacious glimmer. They have spilled from beds of rocks banked around saplings between parked cars. One pebble here. One pebble there. A halting trail, leading somewhere. I walk the same circles knowing I am not circling at all.

4:00 p.m. There are now 438 cases linked to the Smithfield plant alone. Sioux Falls is home to the second-hottest COVID spot in the nation, according to national news reports. Go team! We have surpassed the Cook County Jail in Chicago; are behind only the USS *Theodore Roosevelt*. By this time today the governor has rejected Mayor TenHaken's request for a blanket shelter-in-place order, citing as her big reason: "science, facts, and data." She also has rejected his request that the state set up an isolation center for families of Smithfield workers.

5:00 p.m. Announcement that the CDC is sending a team to examine the Smithfield plant. I know what I would say to an official of the CDC if I bumped into one. I'd tell Harry, Mary, and Jane to check out also the small cinder-block casinos that line the city streets, adjoined to bars, adjoined to gas stations—freestanding incubators.

"Can he take it with applesauce?" Nurse G asks a caller who is having trouble getting a Missouri patient to keep medicine down.

"My new friend in 32 still has his jeans on," notes Nurse E about a patient she's seen with the camera. Though very sick, he refuses to take off his favorite jeans.

6:00 p.m. On the ABC evening news flashes the set face of Governor Noem, the pleading face of the mayor, their stand-off detailed by anchor David Muir. South Dakotans are always shocked when the state receives national attention. I wonder if the coverage will jar loose stuck notions about the state's relation to the pandemic.

7:00 p.m. The light is late but still strong after I clock out. It glistens on icy parking-lot edges. As the social fabric tatters, as various systems struggle and war, there are more and more conundrums, and with them more need to find a way to "be" amid disarray. I think of how, at fifty-six, I was recently carded when in line to buy a bottle of wine to go with dinner. I think of how another clerk, in her seventies, behind the Kwik Stop counter, commented: "You have pretty hair. You do." I think of the advice I got at Ace Hardware when buying wood to burn in the fireplace after our basement boiler conked out: "Did you know you can start a fire with stale popcorn? Or chicken skin?" I didn't.

April 16–17
Never Forget Agustín Rodríguez

7:00 p.m. Earlier in the day the Smithfield plant became the number one U.S. hot spot with 518 positive employee tests and another 126 cases of infection connected to the facility of sooty bricks and white chutes, located next to the brown Big Sioux River and quite near downtown Sioux Falls with its upscale boutiques and loft apartments, some selling (at least before the pandemic) for more than a million dollars. A team from the CDC has arrived to tour the plant and formulate a checklist of actions that need to occur before reopening can be considered.

On my drive to work I think of my partner back at our cold home on the edge of downtown. The boiler is still busted. Last night the temperature outside dipped well under thirty degrees. One thing is certain, this day will end as it began—with one of us feeding the fireplace wood after shoveling ashes. When shoveling ashes a cloud engulfs your leaning head and you sip dust, taste dust, a surprisingly neutral flavor.

8:00 p.m. Wearing a mask is now mandatory in the telehealth building. I strap on my favorite of the two effective masks Brooklyn has provided me with. Cloth stretches over facial features like dough set out to rise. Eyeframe lenses are steamed up before I reach the unit. Arriving, I ask Nurse V, nearly forty years of experience, what to do about that. She always has answers. She suggests I wipe lenses with shaving cream before I report to my next shift. The secretary I am taking over for tells me that handling phone calls is almost impossible with a thick fabric mask in place. She advises that I pull down my mask with one hand as I pick up the phone with the other.

Five of the eight COVID patients in the local ICU are people of color. Seven are participating in a trial run by Mayo Clinic that involves transfusing plasma from recovered COVID patients who have antibodies against the virus. Some are simultaneously being given the controversial hydroxychloroquine treatment, although within the week labor leaders will instruct Smithfield workers to stop taking the drug, citing studies that it actually raises the death rate from COVID.

9:00 p.m. My other coworker tonight, Nurse J, is the one who during my last shift was working bedside. He turns and through his pale-blue surgical mask lets me know he has received a letter from our hospital organization informing him he was exposed to the virus. I assume he means email message. I wait for the rest. Nurse J is one of my favorite nurses because of his dry sense of humor. I wait to hear that he is joking. But it is not a joke: the silence that follows the admission tells me that. His presence here tells me that he has not been required to quarantine, and if he was required to tell our supervisors it did not matter. When scary events occur I can disassociate with ease. I mastered the skill young: a method of surviving abuse. Delayed reaction to bad stuff: poker face first, terror and pain second. Once I passed an Iowa school physical exam while nursing a fractured femur. Once, in Brooklyn, when I had pneumonia, I was judged by a doctor to be a forty-year-old guy with a bit of a cough: not until he examined the X-ray did he see how ill I was, then *I got a letter*—he was embarrassed to call. "Oh," I murmur.

It happens that my partner of thirty years has an autoimmune illness, thus is especially vulnerable to the virus. It happens that we have, Nurse J and I, ten hours left of our shift together in the poorly ventilated hub. Nowhere for fear to go, even if I did let it out out out. A moist dark spot blooms in the middle of the mask that is starting to make my skin itch. "Oh," I say again, only hours later to think: *What if I bring the virus home?* Then, *I make $14.95 an hour. In two and a half years I've worked up to that figure from $12.80, ten cents above the lowest hourly wage*

the hospital pays support specialists. If we get sick, the deductible
is $2,000—more money than I make in an entire month. . . .

10:00 p.m. Settings on ventilators of our COVID patients at
various sites were adjusted earlier. Nothing more will be heard
from them unless there is a crisis. Sedated, they sleep. There
is no further talk about Nurse J's exposure or anything else.
Seated, the two nurses ply their phones, they yawn. Sioux Falls,
number-one hot spot in the nation, and yawns abound. It is, on
one hand, no mystery. We have a low census hovering at about
fifty patients spread over thirteen sites—low because no elective surgeries are being done and anyone who can avoid it is
not coming to the hospital. And the two have completed initial
camera rounds. Despite the recent noise of technological change
to address a national crisis, many clinical eICU minds remain
configured to function in their traditional fashion. I am witnessing the mainstay rubric for telehealth as it exists in this era of
development. It is lists of names, columns of data to be swept
through: Kafka and Microsoft. It does not scamper to the rescue
unless an alarm sounds, and even then the first thing to do is
get the bedside providers busy doing their job. The eICU most
usually serves as a valuable double check. It is Socratic: treatment via questions nurses ask one another and ask the doctor on
duty. It has an academic tilt. It distributes hundreds of iPads to
old exhausted nurses and young inexperienced nurses at far-flung
sites (Scotland, South Dakota!) that might not ever be used, since
in a panic you—young or old—do not try new things that might
cost a life. It installs the River Lethe Machine everyone in the
unit hopes they will never have to touch. No waiting room exists
here to be besieged by the dry cough and the fever. One phone
line can receive only one call at a time. There are a limited number of beds at each site that cameras and mics and iPads could
cover, and many sites, a great many, had to request help specifically even for the designated beds. Do it by pushing a button in

the room or by calling me. Patients were filtered out constantly, as opposed to filtered in, due to cost considerations and other reasons, like the vile tendency of certain physicians to refuse to work with our excellent telehealth female doctors. Why had I thought it would be different tonight? I knew why the air was stale with lethargy, with night-shift stamina challenges of mental numbness and eyestrain and blood-sugar undulations, but to experience this institutional calm as the storm hits feels surreal. I am getting angry at the situation—at the helplessness of everyone. The willingness to look away, to ignore.

11:00 p.m. On the wall TV screen flashes the worried face of Kooper Caraway, president of the Sioux Falls AFL-CIO chapter. He represents Smithfield workers. He claims concerns about the plant's safety were expressed (we're watching the transcription scroll) six weeks ago, before the company offered workers that $500 "responsibility bonus" if they did not miss a day in April, the month of Easter, the month of the highest ham sales. He goes on to say that Governor Noem's refusal to agree to the request of the mayor for an isolation center would "make Ayn Rand blush." The state's leader suggested that anyone who wanted to could quarantine at a hotel! For a cost, of course! He cites her refusal to put a halt on evictions and utility cutoffs. Without running water, no hygiene, but no sir, there will be no halt on cutoffs.

Nurse J—the citizen who, in my opinion, has just been screwed over by the hospital organization he works for—has an additional thing to say at last. He laments, after the report is over: "But what could the state have done?" For a lifetime this loyal nurse has lived in the state, and that's the idea of the state that the state, in the end, has encouraged citizens to form. No state taxes here. No car inspections and plenty of vehicles on the street without bumpers or with garbage bags for windows. Scant environmental oversight, which created the opportunity for the Big Sioux River to become the thirteenth-most-polluted body of water in the nation. The state can't do anything. It's not its job to do. But in doing nothing it does do something to itself.

12:00 a.m. Over eighty languages are spoken by Smithfield plant workers. Spanish speakers and speakers of Nepalese predominate. To aid with the translation process there are a limited number of monitors that can be wheeled into rooms at the main hospital. A translator is then dialed up to help. The protocol is cumbersome, however, and two nurses got together in their free time to address the problem, creating a Spanish cheat sheet they laminated, placed in each ICU room. Nurse J offers to show me a copy. Leaning away from his reach as he leans away from my reach, I somehow get the copy.

> I am your nurse. *Soy su enfermera.*
> Are you short of breath? *¿Tienes problemas para respirar?*
> Can you squeeze my hand? *¿Puede apretar mi mano?*
> You are okay. *Está bien.*
> Your family loves you. *Su familia le ama.*
> We are going to remove your breathing tube because you
>   no longer need it. *Vamos a remover el tubo porque no lo*
>   *necesita más.*

1:00 a.m. Dr. R, in India, who knows I have New York City connections, calls to ask me how my friends and family are doing there. I update him. He tells me about COVID eliminating a young Manhattan medical student in the middle of his residency.

2:00 a.m. Sitting in the unit is the mason jar full of homemade sanitizer the previous nurse brewed and left for our use. It has the consistency of water. It is peppermint scented.

"Oh no," rumbles Nurse V. There has been a mistake at Site 10. Two doctors ordered the same blood-pressure medication for the same patient, and a nurse gave all the medication at once. The patient's blood pressure has plunged. He needs a "presser" now to raise the heartbeat. One drug leads to another. Kidneys, watch out.

3:00 a.m. Walk my three laps in the dark parking lot. It is cold. I think of a retired history of science professor in a nursing home in the Bronx where a number of residents have died of the virus. An old friend of Anne's family. In Brooklyn Heights, we dined many times with Tom Settle and his wife Dorothy James—a German professor at Hunter. Tom's specialty was Galileo. Looking at the stars tonight I miss his wit. I think of his glass of ice and scotch tilted in one direction, his smile tilted in another. For years he taught at Polytechnic Institute of Brooklyn. An admiral's son. His rare books went to Columbia University. He used to spend part of every year in Florence. Dorothy had published short stories in handsome slicks like *Redbook* and *Mademoiselle* in the early 1970s. She was the person who gave Anne, at fourteen, her best piece of writing advice. "It's so easy to let it go," Dorothy warned, and Anne listened.

4:00 a.m. An alert sounds: boing boing boing. A nurse at Site 12 is calling in distress: "I've been fighting this [vented] guy for almost an hour. The Precedex is just not settling him down— he's going to self-extubate if we don't do something fast. Can we get a fentanyl push?" Nurse V gets her the order from the doctor. Patient down.

5:00 a.m. At Site 18 the patient who drank two bottles of cough syrup leaves against medical advice. At Site 6 arrives an inebriated man who fell hands first into a fire pit with predictable results. Another Smithfield patient enters the Sioux Falls ICU from ER. Forty years old. Hypertension caused by the virus is not responding to medication. Our nurses have noticed a tendency for the heart rate of COVID sufferers to spike.

Information about the first Smithfield fatality—the one who died right before noon during my last shift—has hit the national news. A church-attending, sixty-four-year-old man: Agustín Rodríguez.

Born in El Salvador, he worked in the factory's Cut Department for almost twenty years. Ill with fever, he went to work anyway with the hope of earning the April "responsibility bonus." His wife, Angelita, has this to say in the Sioux Falls *Argus Leader*: "I lost him because of that horrible place. Those horrible people and their supervisors, they're sitting in their homes and they're happy with their families. In the name of Jesus Christ, these people need to face justice."

In the Upper Midwest, because of meat-processing-plant closures, the farmers are now stuck with animals at finishing weight, and no buyers. Piglets will have to be shot or suffocated because there is no room for them to develop in the hog barns. Out on the East Coast, due to Quarantine Loneliness Syndrome, reports indicate animal shelters are running low on cats and dogs and other strays needing adoption.

6:00 a.m. Read company email announcing furloughs to stem the financial losses caused by pandemic preparation. Hundreds of medical workers are waking up (if they slept) without an income. Hundreds of factory workers are waking and wondering if they are sick or experiencing definitive symptoms. What to do? Few test sites. Closed clinics. The health system that invented the eICU had also created a telehealth app to support virtual office visits, but access to the necessary technology is not a given in this low-wage region.

7:00 a.m. I clock out. I leave behind the drone of sleepy nurses giving reports to other sleepy nurses. At the end of the line of stations I shuffle to the right, passing the posted number—in the thousands—of lives purportedly saved by the eICU since its inception more than fifteen years before. It was derived from data captured by the unit while treating patients—respiratory data and the all-important Glasgow Coma Score, among other figures. The way I understood it, the dire test results of eICU survivors were compared to the outcomes of other ICU patients with the same test results but not benefitting from the extra layer of tele-health clinical support. A few nurses joked about the tabulation equation. The gist: the numbers were iffy. The numbers were, and were not, human beings.

I get in my car. A satellite somewhere allows me to consult my phone. I find the latest songs my friend Ivan has dispatched to me on his commute to PNC bank on Seventh Avenue. Lee Konitz's "I'll Remember April." (Konitz died of COVID April 15 at Lenox Hill Hospital.) Harvey and the Moonglows doing "Mama Loochie." I have come to think of Ivan as the last security guard standing, his beard and copious smile and the bob in his step protecting it all—Manhattan to Brooklyn to Queens to the Bronx to Staten Island, and me too. I need each of these notes, sweet downpours to dilute sour echoes as I sit in the parking lot of the killdeer, waiting to calm down, drive on.

Well, maybe it won't hit us hard out here. We're South Dakota. The wish. *Ben, I was exposed.* The reality is the virus may have walked into our unit without facing any urgent, effec-tive resistance. The telehealth facility "lockdown" had completely failed in this case—if its aim was to prevent any employees from being placed in high-risk situations.

It's the lifestyle of those workers—that's to blame. But couldn't the same dead-wrong thing be said of Nurse J? That it was his South Dakota–cowboy cultural attitude that got him exposed on the floor and caused him to report to work last night untested for COVID, ready for action. When, of course, the managers of the health organization we worked for were ultimately respon-sible for workplace safety, just as the Smithfield management team was ultimately responsible for the gigantic factory with few entrances and the elbow-to-elbow production lines and for the decision, at the outbreak's start, to post COVID-19 warnings only in English when dozens of languages were spoken in the locker rooms and on the floors. (On April 20, BuzzFeed News would publish a statement by a Smithfield representative blaming the outbreak on "living circumstances in certain cultures.")

Smithfield had offered workers the $500 "responsibility bonus" to boost attendance during a frightening time. Our employer had recently announced a $500 "relief payment" to salaried and hourly employees. There was no attendance stipulation, thank goodness. But given the dedication of most nurses maybe that could be left unsaid. Turning the key in the ignition I notice a nurse who had reported minutes ago has fled the building, surgical mask dangling from her fingers. She needs air already. Did Nurse J tell her about his exposure? What would she do? For herself, her large family? She was the best of the best nurses.

I wave. I speed away.

A wretched and hapless shift, except for the genius of that translation cheat sheet crafted by two young nurses doing a good job under roughest circumstances. It was more effective, and practical, than the high-tech options. A solution with 100 percent reliability. No connectivity issues, software glitches. No snarls of cords. No username and password prompts. That sheet defined the essence of good care: an affordable idea applicable across a broad patient population, and, equally as important, infused with tenderness no healing process could be complete without.

Are you having pain? *¿Tienes dolor?*
Are you short of breath? *¿Tienes problemas para respirar?*
You are safe. *Está seguro/a.* (male/female pt)
We are going to take good care of you. *Vamos a cuidarle muy bien.*

LOG 2

The Magic of Palm Place

*. . . listen for one's own deepest, most authentic music,
no matter how discordant it may sound, and let it rip.*
—Stephen Kessler, "Bukowski:
The Long View"

May–October 2020
Locking Three Doors

Holding the wrong day job at exactly the wrong time was not a
new phenomenon in my working life. In October of 1987, when
the stock market crashed, I was a graduate student employed in
the New York Stock Exchange Library, which instantly became
an internal data hub of the crisis, we clerks (happily owning not
one share of stock) charged with manually gathering and feeding
ticker numbers to managers to feed to the media besieging the
brass doors of the Exchange at 11 Wall. During the *Satanic Verses*
controversy—when phoned bomb threats targeted stores selling
the novel by Salman Rushdie—I happened to be a bag checker
at Remsen Books in Brooklyn Heights, and upon being handed
each bag wondered if it might blow me, and my writing dreams,
sky high. On September 11, 2001, I was the first clerk to report to
a Manhattan skyscraper suite and from a window saw the second
plane hit the World Trade Center at 9:03 a.m. Yet again luck held.

When we were evacuating, my Seventh Avenue address spared me from being choked by the toxic ash falling towers spewed.

Having navigated these situations, I hoped to handle the fate of being a secretary in a telehealth ICU unit as the pandemic commenced. After all, I was no health care hero treating patients at personal risk. I was helper to the helpers, the eICU nurses in a windowless hub with the ambiance of a cyber-equipped submarine designed to glide through Midwest soil, under parking lots. If within harrowing earshot and screen view of patients as the crisis played out at hospitals the unit supported, I bore no responsibility for outcomes. I was the phone-cradling traffic controller. List minder. Brewer of calming peppermint tea for the staff, mixer of Virgin Marys to enliven glum holiday shifts. Succeeding during each twelve-hour stint merely meant arriving on time, in a supportive mood, and executing straightforward tasks I knew well after more than two years of service. I'd be there for my team, I would.

I had a perfect attendance record and good reviews during that employment period in South Dakota's most disruptive space: its largest city, the cement prairie, where two large regional health systems are headquartered. I was, then, as astonished as my supervisor, when after that April 16–17 night shift I did not return for another.

Six weeks of the pandemic was all it had taken for a symphony of terrors to build incrementally to an abrupt climax. I woke in tears. I found that I dreaded the rhythmic wheeze of ventilators that filled the unit—dreaded having to discharge another Smithfield factory worker not to HOME but to DEATH in the eCare Manager census system—dreaded the attitudes of a few staff members, so worn out from having dealt for years with comas caused by diabetic ketoacidosis and half-failed suicide attempts and fentanyl ODs and the I-90 car crash victims that they could, well, hardly be bothered to take another disaster seriously. I heard more than one nurse insist, "We're all going to get it," as Lenny Bruce, at the height of the Cold War, opined, "We're all gonna die."

If not ready to fail coworkers, I was much less ready to be harmed at fifty-six by a work environment increasingly out of control (funny how growing older can make you less and less ready to die). When the tears stopped, I called my supervisor on the chance that he would be able to provide safety assurances. I said: "I think the virus is likely to get into the unit. Do you?" The answer: "Probably . . . it probably will." Nothing else. I hung up.

Turns out this was a new kind of workplace crisis for me. Though I did not bear the burden of patient care, I was hardly a nameless functionary as at Remsen Books and the NYSE. No, the first voice a small-town doctor with a crashing patient heard when calling for telehealth assistance was mine. *"Support Specialist Ben. How can I help you?"* But perhaps the most significant factor in my breakdown was the fact I was experiencing the calamity not in New York—where my good luck outweighed the bad—but in the Midwest, where I had barely escaped a dangerous family situation before landing at New York University at age twenty-two. As I had tried to tough it out during the first weeks of the pandemic—as I told myself what the hardy nurses told themselves: *You've got this!*—each shift raised my panic and fear level slowly but steadily, in such a way that I possessed no full awareness I was so near a breaking point. With sinister efficiency the nightmare of the Present had begun colluding with the Past, and finally new terrors danced with old.

After fleeing the eICU, I quickly took two unprecedented (for me) actions. I applied for medical leave and for unemployment benefits to help make ends meet while I figured things out. The leave was approved promptly. When more than six weeks went by without my receiving a decision from the state of South Dakota about the unemployment application, I was forced to cash in a

401K plan connected to the data-vetting job I had held at a business called Infobase in New York City.

As months went by, Anne and I lived off savings (and then the benefits, which did finally get approved, in less than two hours, after I elicited the help of State Senator Reynold Nesiba, who contacted Secretary of Labor Marcia Hultman directly).

I extended the medical leave twice so that I could receive more treatment from the trauma specialist whose letter, thanks to protections provided employees by the Americans with Disabilities Act (ADA), prevented me from being fired.

> [My client] has a diagnosis of Post-Traumatic Stress Disorder with an extensive childhood history of multiple traumas. One of the primary difficulties that the past trauma has created [is] a distrust of institutions, which should have protected him [schools, public clinics] and did not. Unfortunately, this has contributed to Ben being away from his position since late April following a night shift when a nurse who had just been exposed to the COVID virus was allowed to work in the unit, not only exposing Ben to danger but his spouse who has an underlying medical condition.
>
> I would ask that . . . Ben be allowed to transfer within the system to a similar job with similar pay.

Here's how it can be with such a case of complex PTSD:

You lock the porch door to keep the danger out. You lock the next door. You lock the third door to the house. But still not feeling safe, you must keep alert, ready to dive for cover, because ten or fifteen or even twenty times a day you imagine gunshots from a passing car shattering window glass and hitting you and your partner of thirty-one years, the poet. Or on a walk around the block on a quiet sunny June day you envision a figure running up behind you and planting a knife in your back. Or when you glance over neighbor Judy's fence you see the arm of a corpse stretching across the stoop, fingers curled and still. Or when working in your community garden plot it is vital to keep gardening tools *inside* the fence to prevent a passerby from picking up a hoe and hacking you to death.

Eventually, of course, it was either reenter the workforce or apply for SSI (Supplemental Security Income), which did not seem appropriate. I was definitely wounded, rearranged . . . but disabled to the point of not being able to hold a job? Throughout adulthood I had been jerry-rigging together effective modes of functioning in a wide-range of situations.

In October I began, with the aid of the health system's Human Resources Department, interviewing for new positions. At interviews I described my skill set as "accuracy, consistency, congeniality." After many WebEx interviews I finally got an offer, one I was happy about. It was my first position in Sioux Falls that paid over $15 an hour. The circumstances seemed as safe as anything I could possibly find: no contact with the public and a desk of my own—the first since my desk in Byerly Hall in Cambridge during a Cinderella year of experimentation at Harvard's Radcliffe Institute. Title: Centralized Scheduling Specialist. Responsibility: booking appointments for diagnostic tests over the phone. Location: Palm Place, near the airport.

No working nights or holidays. Eight-hour shifts. After a year I'd have the option of working from home, a rare privilege here, even during COVID. There had been over 600 deaths in South Dakota to this point. More than 1,000 new infections were being reported daily in a state with fewer than 900,000 citizens.

First days at jobs were all the same and all different. You started out knowing nothing, the newbie in the center of an awkward swirl of attention. You started as the one that the others did not quite trust or could not quite place. You had no idea who knew what about you—how deeply the trickle of the resume info had penetrated the department, or how it had been conveyed. There'd be whispers of things the staff thought you too soft to hear and whispers about things they did not want Newbie to know right away or did not know how to address with Newbie, not knowing Newbie. Your first day on the job was like being the youngest child in the family: welcomed, flattered, examined, deceived.

The different thing here? I was not coming into the situation at full strength.

It was akin to being sent behind front lines to heal, only the war was still in me.

November 18
"I'm Over It!"

On the fourteen-minute drive to Palm Place I pass a Minnesota Avenue billboard reading SACRED HEART OF JESUS HAVE MERCY ON US, then the Crack'd Pot (Since 1974) family restaurant, known for homemade soups and rhubarb pies, affordable strip steaks, and, most recently, masked employees, a 50 percent occupancy policy, furniture and condiment bottles sanitized with the disinfectant spray Microban 24. GOD BLESS AMERICA blinks the sign outside, letters early-digital-age dot-matrix orange. Across the railroad tracks the airport named after World War II fighter pilot Joe Foss is being expanded by bulldozers that have cleared acres next to the existing tarmac, a yawn of dirt that makes it look as if a 747 had just been buried there.

After parking where an orchard used to be, I decide not to double-mask. I snap on one pale blue mask, just one, to keep my lenses from steaming up, and to help my new coworkers hear what I say. *It's all about building relationships.* Then I cross the lot carrying a backpack containing a box of fifty more masks, a pale green bud vase, boxes of tea, and a few postcards to pin up in my cube: the Charles River and the Grand Central Oyster Bar.

Having no new company photo-ID badge yet, I knock on the electronically secure glass door to get the attention of the receptionist. Inside is 1980s IBM tan; the sprawling facade is brown mall with pebbled walls and a few cantilevered pseudo–Frank Lloyd Wright touches. As I enter, no potted palms do I see. Rather, there is a stalk topped with the computer screen with the job of taking the temps of entering employees. Next to it is a table offering a strip of adhesive yellow dots. From my last pandemic position, I know that after I am screened I must apply today's color dot to my person to prove to others I am not feverish. And masks. Plenty of masks. I'm comforted this health system is now making masks freely available: it was not the case last spring.

Quick I lean toward the screen, fitting my head into the green outline of a head. "Success!" a robotic voice exclaims. Then, as instructed, I take a seat in a puffy lobby chair to wait for my "Orientation Ambassador" to appear, careful not to touch the arms of the chair. For more than six months Anne and I have avoided public places. The prospect of COVID-19 heightens the meaning of every action I take now. I need to summon extra concentration to stay safe.

"Boy you dressed up too much!" quips masked Ambassador on arriving. I wear a button-down and new jeans and now, suddenly, a patina of embarrassment. "Well, . . ." I mumble. "You'll learn fast!" she quips. "Before we go to the department I'll give you a tour!" Red haired and slight, she wears old jeans, an unbuttoned, untucked flannel shirt over a T-shirt out of a folk song.

Windowless hall. Ambassador points out stairs leading to a second level not worth visiting and a cafeteria that is. I note the cafeteria has a complex identity. One sign reads: The Frond Café.

Another sign reads: The Old Orchard Café. They, the café, consists of a grill behind a short tray rail, coffee-drink apparatus, cooler cases of cola, hanging trees of salty snacks, and a square, large seating area surrounded by tinted windows that lend the parking lot an artichoke hue. I immediately decide not to eat there, however, because I see four undistanced, unmasked male employees poking breakfast items with plastic forks, looking in no mood to adapt.

"NowI'lltakeyoutoScheduling!" announces Ambassador. I hear she is almost as nervous as I am. Why? We turn left, right, less tan, more gray, and there I stand, inhaling in a department of cubicles scrunched under a ceiling six feet lower than the lobby's ceiling. Three cubes on each side of an aisle leading to other departments. "That cube is yours!" Ambassador pipes. But not mine quite yet, still occupied by another worker's plastic flowers, 2020 dog calendar, stuffed pooch toy. "There's a lot of cleaning up to do around here!" she adds in oblique and flustered explanation. I nod. I don't make things worse for her. I doubt it is her fault, whatever it is that is wrong.

I take another irritated look at doggy cube. I wanted to see a place cleared for me. It's no time to have no personal space to sanitize and make safe. Directly above the desk chair is a circular ceiling vent rimmed by dangling snippets of duct tape that, thank goodness, failed to seal it. Air flow is a crucial element of workplace safety now.

"Pull that chair into my cube." I obey. Ambassador's cube is open on one side, so the scheduler in the next cube can tap her on the shoulder if need be. That black-haired worker is unmasked like the others I've seen at desks. I remain in the aisle as we exchange greetings. She tells me she used to work as a nurse in Scotland, South Dakota. I know the town. The eICU supported the staff at its minuscule hospital. From across the aisle comes a burst of scheduler-speak. "Aw sugar butt! Send that one to ASH."

"You stinkpot! ASH is full!" "Awesome sauce! No ASH for her then!"

"Ash?" I ask. Ambassador flutters as she answers. "We use. . . ." I hear the next word as "new-moan-icks." I don't get it. Then do. *Mnemonics*—systems designed to aid memory. A virus of acronyms. "See ASH means Area Specialty Hospital. A-S-H." "Okay." (Coincidence: often at the eICU I worked with a Seattle-based Dr. Ashwin who insisted we call him Ash.) "It'll take you six months to get a handle on things." "Oh." "That's completely normal. Barbara, our manager, isn't in today, or I'd introduce you." ABB. Absent Boss Barbara. "Her boss is Nadine." BBN. Big Boss Nadine.

Above Ambassador's bobbing head is a shelf lined with personal items. Son's high-school-graduation photo. Daughter in a tutu. The letters BELIEVE cut out of wood. The gift shop at the main hospital sells inspirational items like this to employees.

She relates a story about her boy. He was a wonderful baseball player until age twelve when he struck out to end a playoff game and decided he never wanted to have that feeling again and quit cold. She laughs her scared laugh. She says she is a former ICU nurse. Did that for eight years before transferring here.

Into my hand she presses a thick binder of department protocols. I open it, page through, and get dizzier. Most of the inserts are in nine-point type. Next she hands me what? It's black. Plastic. A gaunt half-circle . . . like a tiara designed by Kafka. One end is ornamented with a disc. "Your headset. I'll put you on mute so you only hear calls."

I admit I've never donned a phone headset. She instructs, and cheers me on—her new boy—until my scalp is harnessed. "Good job!" She yanks down her mask to take a gulp of coffee, as I push my chair away from her lips, her nose, her air. Safer. She fixes the mask. I wheel my chair forward. I decide never to take off my mask in this department. To go somewhere else to quaff my coffee or water or cyanide.

In the corner of her screen is a square window that allows her to manage the phone. There are options. One of them is WORK. One of them is READY. She tells me that when she is on WORK the phone won't ring. "See, I'm still on WORK." I see. "Well, want to start?" I place a spiral notebook on the binder. Already there is one note: *ASH = Area Specialty Hospital.* She clicks READY and it happens. A new health care world pours into my ear, a cadence of weary or snippy or laconic clinic-nurse test requests and Ambassador's harried responses as she races through the scheduling software screens to locate appointment choices. Her shoe never stops tapping.

First she reschedules an MRI for a meatpacking-plant employee who does not speak English and had been previously slotted for a machine in the hospital basement, but that won't work because there are not enough translators available on that day to book one, meaning that the internet translating service called MARTTI (My Accessible Real-Time Trusted Interpreter) must be used . . . and the walls of the basement are too thick to allow the internet signal through.

I'm jarred by another coincidence. The new job is starting where the last ended, with dire communication issues: Hispanic employees from Smithfield meatpacking plant filling hospital beds after getting infected with COVID, and English-speaking ICU nurses and doctors using cheat sheets in the struggle to communicate with family members.

Appointment rescheduled, Ambassador leaves herself on WORK and turns to explain: "Each exchange should last no more than two minutes. Confirm patient name and birthday and weight and allergy status, time and place of the test, and other things, depending on the test: CT (computed tomography scan) or MRI or ultrasound or DEXA (bone density scan). Give the nurse the prep instructions to give the patient. After hanging up, finish booking the transaction in the system as swiftly as possible, making sure that it is married to the doctor's faxed or electronic order. Then put yourself on READY again." I grimace. No listening to music as in the eICU while I enter patient lab data into the virtual chart. No WBGO, WKCR, WQXR. . . . "Time and call-volume statistics for each scheduler are cited in a weekly department email. A good review depends on them. We take over 400 calls some days. The team on any given shift consists of between five and nine schedulers, some working from home."

The long ago December I worked as a Santa at the Herald Square Macy's store, I was supposed to place a child on my lap every sixty seconds, but there was no timer in the blinking Santaland hut, just a slouching, unconcerned elf in revealing tights. At the eICU I was always racing against the clock to keep up with census management and charting, but, again, no timer existed. Odd that here, in a nonemergency setting, there should be such a wild rush. Or maybe not so odd, given that these tests cost thousands of dollars, keep the hospital solvent.

On READY again, more voices pour in, as I shadow, scribbling whatever I can absorb as Ambassador click-click-clicks to keep her statistics respectable. "That time is too early at ASH—patient is coming all the way from Chancellor—let's do it at Sixty-ninth and Marion." "MRI of the brain with and without contrast on Tuesday, December. . . ." "Need a venous duplex left lower extremity. When's the soonest you can get the patient in?" "Visual swallow studies are only done on Thursday." "MRI with arthrogram." "How much does the patient weigh? That machine has a weight limit of 450." "Eighty-five and just getting her first bone scan! That's an achievement." "Lori from the vein clinic on Louise." "Jada from the county jail. . . ." "Patient can't make it for the MRI on the twentieth because he was just diagnosed with COVID." "She can't make her appointment because her husband is in the VA with COVID." "We'll have to cancel Johnson's CT on the fourth because he was just diagnosed with COVID."

In the midst of the action, around noon, we hear sniffling in the next cube that turns into a moan that turns into a half-stifled wail. "I'm over it!" Ambassador gets up and, out of my hearing, talks to her distressed coworker. When the two return to their places, one of the schedulers across the aisle gets up and pulls Ambassador aside. When their private conference ends, Ambassador puts herself on READY again, but I can see she is not.

"Gena from the Dizzy Clinic." "Two prisoners need IVs when the mobile unit visits the penitentiary next week." "Ultrasounds are hard to come by on that day." "At 8:30 start drinking contrast for the 9:30 CT." "Are you seeing a lot of COVID reschedules? When the screenings slow down, the cancers are caught later, and the outcomes change." "Internal derangement of the right knee, seventeen years old." "I'm a teacher scheduled for a liver test, but given COVID and the lack of subs I can't get the day off and need to reschedule for Christmas week—I won't be working then."

Next up is a call from the retired machinist who needs an MRI lumbar scan to check for radiculopathy (pinched nerves in the spinal column), but he might have metal in his eyes so he needs to have an X-ray scheduled *before* the MRI to rule out the possibility. An MRI magnet will pull metal out of the body. Shavings could shred his retinas.

The scheduler in the next cube quietly weeps during long breaks between the few calls she answers. Hunched over her desktop four feet behind my increasingly hunched back, she keeps muttering, "I'm over it." I don't get it. In the middle of the afternoon she begins sneezing and coughing and cries even louder: "I'm over it!"

I don't find out what "it" is until right before the shift is over. Ambassador, blushing, whispers, "Sandy's live-in boyfriend Jaydon called her late in the morning to say he had tested positive for COVID." And there was no one in the department on this day invested with enough authority to compel the departure of the magical thinker.

After the shift, sitting in a car in the parking lot, I call Anne. "I can't believe it," I stammer. "The first day. What do we do?" It's a twenty-minute talk, and not too focused, as we are in shock. I say many things, but do not tell her I was wearing only one mask, as I don't want to scare her more, and, frankly, I'm ashamed about having underestimated the danger of Palm Place after being an expert at being afraid for months. Eventually, I pull out and enter the traffic flow on Benson. It's dark. Traffic is heavy. Many of those who worked day shifts are not on their way home but on their way to a night job, with fast food in tow, because here many day jobs pay well below $15 an hour. That's nomadism, Sioux Falls style, nothing like a Hollywood script. Two miles one direction, three miles in another, stop, start, stop. A treaded trudge of never getting ahead. The 401K has spared me from a second day job, at least. I was a fool for cashing it in and smart too. It wasn't near enough to retire on anyway.

When I pull into our driveway off West Tenth Street, the phone rings. Anne and I talk for another twenty minutes as I stare at the door of the old-style cottage garage. We decide on the most cautious course of action, given the fact that Anne is on an immunosuppressant medication, making her especially vulnerable to the virus. Fourteen days of masking in the house except when showering. Sleeping in separate bedrooms. Tomorrow I will cancel the Thanksgiving turkey order I placed at the food co-op. Tonight four glasses of white wine are required to begin to calm down.

Still, I can't sleep. I retabulate realities, feel the emotions. I do not want to return to Palm Place but I've got to try again. It's my fourth day job in five years, after we moved here to push forward writing projects connected to the urban Midwest, complex diverse cities that constituted a region within a region that had never been covered in the media in sufficient detail. More than half of South Dakota's residents (not including those who reside on reservations) now lived in such places—drawn by opportunities not available in the fading small towns. Some used a diploma from one of the state universities to make the leap, but most did not need to. Less than 10 percent of Sioux Falls jobs require a college education, and being overqualified does not help. Saved as NEW is the email from the state informing me unemployment benefits have expired. I've used every day of leave the company is required by law to give me. . . . Anne knocks on the wall between us. I knock three times. Our code for *I love you*.

History relates that on this day there were 1,387 new COVID cases in South Dakota and 30 deaths. Over the last week the average has been 1,425 cases a day.

November 19
Krabbenhoft & Co.

Face moist under masks, lenses steamed up, dressed a little less nice, I bow to Temp Scanner, apply pink badge dot, and move on, clutching the bag of desk charms I do not unpack on this morning either, as the cube supposedly mine is still laden with canine memorabilia. "You came back!" exclaims Ambassador in greeting. "The last person we hired was so spooked she left after two days. Not a call or email to let us know!"

I inquire about the status of Magical Thinker, who is not chanting in her cube. I get more of the story. Boyfriend was symptomatic all weekend, had been tested on Monday. MT, who spent the weekend with him, unmasked, in a small house in the suburb of Tea, reported to work on Monday, Tuesday, yesterday. Today she is being tested. "I'm worried," I say. Ambassador confesses concern too.

Her wrist quavers as she slips on her Kafka tiara and hands me mine. But instead of clicking READY and taking calls she talks more. "Well, confusion is normal around here! This afternoon you're going to have to spend time alone studying the binder. I have to work on the six-week schedule for the department." "Fine with me." She looks down at her shoes. She laughs that unhappy laugh again. "You know, a few weeks ago I smelled something bad. I thought another scheduler had tooted. But the smell did not go away. It got stronger. Ha! I guessed another scheduler had had way too much chili for supper, but. . . ." She pointed at her Nikes. "I'd stepped in dog poop—*fresh*!" I like tangents. Truth often is encased in circularities. But whatever was encapsulated here I could not, right then, grasp. . . . I spoke up.

"I'm afraid there's a chance we might have been exposed. The three of us were sitting so close all day yesterday."

"I've been thinking about that. I worked right next to her two days before that."

"I'm not sure I can focus on training today. What should I do?"

"Call Employee Health. See what they say. Do what is right for you and your family."

I leave the department. At the edge of They, the cafeteria, is a short corridor, and in it a secluded ledge looking out on a patio under an overhang. Stacked chairs out there. Thick security bars on the perimeter let in wind that shuffles dry leaves strewn on the cement. Staring at that shadowland, I call Employee Health but can't get through and decide to leave for the day and try again from home. Absent Boss Barbara is not in and present to detain me. Ambassador, I feel, will have no problem with it. I'm right.

"Were the three of you masked?" asks the Employee Health nurse.

"Except when drinking or eating or wiping our noses. But the coworker was symptomatic by the end of the day, and we were all in close quarters for eight hours."

"Why did you call?"

"I want to be tested. My wife has an underlying condition, and. . . ."

"Were you unmasked for longer than fifteen minutes?"

"No."

"Do you have any symptoms?"

"No."

"That does not count as an exposure then. You can return to work."

"I'm cleared?"

"Your supervisor will be notified of this call and expect you to report."

"I can't be tested?"

"Not now, but if anything changes, please call back. COVID can come on fast. I just got a call from a doctor who felt fine yesterday but around two in the morning started shaking. He'll be tested today. He's probably positive."

"So if I feel sick I can call back and have a test."

"No, we don't give tests. You have to call your provider to set up the test, *then* call us to let us know you are *getting* a test."

I have my no-cough, no-test marching orders from the non-profit health system still run by the same order of nuns that started it in the early 1900s in response to a diphtheria epidemic. Workers at the area's other health system, an even larger company, have to deal with the recent comments of their CEO, a nonclinician named Kelby Krabbenhoft, who refuses to wear a mask at work, and who told the *Argus Leader*: "At this point, we feel we've got [COVID] under control. . . . There's not a crisis." Over 10,000 people in South Dakota test positive the week he makes this claim. More than 100 die.

November 21–22
Hello, 1977

Over the weekend Anne and I face each other blue-masked for the logical sake of safety—of preserving the precious marriage that has been a productive and satisfying collaboration on many levels—but the fact is there are spates these crazy days when I no longer feel like the mature writer who, with a trusted companion, returned to learn and grow. I feel as if the roots unearthed are strangling me, making them impossible to study. I feel as if the old madness of domestic fragmentation has hold of me again—is happening all over again.

November 23
Trainer Two

I get back to Palm Place by telling myself, *The worst has happened. Nothing could possibly be as bad as the first day.* I get myself there on the wings of a new strategy to keep safe amid the exposed noses of uncommitted mask wearers. (1) Over the surgical mask wear one of the new antibacterial and deodorizing black Lapcos Live Well face masks I ordered online. (2) When shadowing, touch nothing but pen, Kafka tiara, notebook. (3) Exude much enthusiasm whenever the word "vaccine" is mentioned. (4) When thirsty, tell trainer I need to use restroom and scurry to the Gulp Counter, my new name for that ledge off the cafeteria, and swig while gazing at photos of the New York City marquees that Ivan, loyal friend, has recently sent along. WE'RE IN THIS TOGETHER (King's Theater, the Bronx). LOVE'S IN NEED OF LOVE TODAY, STEVIE WONDER (the Apollo, Harlem).

When green dot and I enter the Scheduling Department I find Magical Thinker is still out, and that Ambassador is missing now also, meaning either that she has tested positive or is even more freaked out by the doings here than me. I do see an unmasked someone seated in the cube I was told was mine. Turns out it is the owner of the canine calendar back from a leave for knee surgery. She sees me and lips peel back from teeth to produce an enigmatic smile. Dark hairdo curls tilting forward, gaze vague, she makes the two vowels of the word she says sound like six vowels: "Weeeel-coooome." She says it twice, as I do not respond the first time, waiting for an acknowledgment of a process that will soon make my desk mine.

As I stand in the aisle, not knowing what to do next, Absent Boss Barbara finally appears and impales me with her full attention. She is short. Broad shoulders, helmet of blond hair. Talking in three-word sentences, she makes every second count. "Big blue stripes! I love it!" Reference to my shirt. "Trainer two today! Right over there!" She doesn't give me time to ask about my desk, scurrying into an unshared office (with a door) that separates INSURANCE REVIEW department from SCHEDULING. T2's cube is across from an unused conference room with a wishful name over the door like all Palm Place meeting rooms: SERENITY.

T2 wears jeans and a lived-in gray hoodie. Her voice is soft and tired. Like Ambassador, she is a single mother with much going on, although I do not learn about any of that until later. I don the Kafka tiara she extends and float to the edge of her domain. I'm thinking about the refrigerated trucks on the Brooklyn waterfront full of hundreds of COVID victims no family member has claimed or a family cannot afford to bury. I'm squinting at the scheduling software over her shoulder and desiring a special device for safe shadowing in COVID Times, a Six-Foot-O-Scope to view what T2 types in the many fields on the many pea-green screens she clicks through after she gets a call requesting a "CT of the chest at Plaza 2 on the Main Campus."

A Gary from Pipestone, Minnesota, checks in to cancel a biopsy because he just had a positive COVID test. His ill voice crackles like fire. A Gene from Rock Rapids, Iowa, wants to reschedule his swallow study because the weather will be iffy tomorrow. His knees are bad. He's afraid of slipping on icy pavement. A clinic nurse phones to book a pneumogram sleep study for a two-year-old. Another clinic nurse demands T2 add a sedation order to an existing MRI of the brain for a one-year-old . . . and I see the whale of a machine swallowing that little limp figure as parents wait, worrying.

Though I had to deal with six different types of EMR (electronic medical record) programs in the eICU, I usually did not have to drill too far into them to reach lab results. It's different with the single scheduling program. In order to book one test, T2 must click through twelve screens. The next booking I lose count after twenty screens. "Any questions?" she asks. There are so many I can think of only one. "How many of each diagnostic machine are there? The main ones?" She says there are five MRI machines and six CT machines and four ultrasound machines.

Between calls T2 tries to give me good news: Absent Boss Barbara is working on getting me access to some phone program called Finesse. From overheard department chatter I learn I have not yet met the person to fear most. That person is Donna, who comes in here not often, being stationed most of the time in Radiology. Every place I've ever worked there has always been at least one person who makes it their job to hassle coworkers. When at Macy's it was the pacing, chain-smoking, wisecracking Santa terrorizer by the name of Mr. Lampe in the charcoal suit.

"Should I book it 'tap dry, no albumin' or what?" yodels a scheduler to the rest of the group. "That's right, Missy!" is T2's reply. A third voice chimes in, drawing the big laugh: "Fake it to make it, Missy!" I heard the title "Missy" last week also. I'm understanding that to be called Missy you need to be very confused and in need of assistance. Will I get called Missy soon? At the eICU I was often included in the category of "ladies"—as when a passing employee shouted "Hello, ladies!" without looking into the unit first. I and They, the cafeteria, should have a talk about this.

How to fit in here, with this particular group of set-in-their-ways schedulers, other than vanish? That oldest trick of mine? At the eICU I noticed how often nurses traipsed to the back of the stifling ochre hub to pound an old pump bottle, treating their hands to shots of lotion, and was moved to invent a lotion bar, actually two, and made signs: LAST CHANCE LOTION BAR / SILVER MOON LOTION BAR. Donations of moisturizing hooch created quite a stock. The expanding display was always good for a laugh even on the worst days when patients coded and the machines tolled. Laughter finished building the bridge imagination started.

After another barrage of virus-related MRI cancellations T2 turns to me at cube's edge, mutters: "South Dakota is the new New York." Four employees at the Pierre, South Dakota, scheduling office have tested positive and it will close for the time being.

On my break I try to start establishing a relationship with the parking lot by looking, listening, drawing connections. The lot ends where a large vacant overgrown lot begins. I walk toward that fringe of emptiness, past ash trees wearing quarter-sized tin medallions indicating inoculation against the Asian longhorned beetle scourge. There is one on a tree in our backyard. It reads: *Arborjet Tree Injection 85733 Arborjet.com.* In the distance flutters the city's biggest American flag, planted by the Camping World RV dealer next to Interstate 90. It is much wider and taller than a Brooklyn brownstone. Gusts make it look like a giant, flexing, red-white-and-blue bicep. That wind blows unhatched robin eggs out of nests in the neighborhood where we live. I have a collection of them. I spot another walker across the lot in a black coat, swinging arms toy-soldier fashion. I hear no song-birds. A few crows slouch on bare branches. There are no cattail ditches nearby, which could explain the lack of certain animals and birds—burrowing rabbits, for example—but the total lack of squirrels and songbirds is odd.

November 24
Daily Prayers

On the drive in, listening to 1010 WINS ("You give us twenty-two minutes, we'll give you the world"), I learn a COVID field hospital is being set up in the borough of Staten Island to handle a surge. The good New York City news is that Astor Place Hairstylists—sometimes referred to as "the United Nations of hair cutting," due to the many different languages spoken by hair stylists—has been saved from extinction by a group of investors that includes former mayor Michael Bloomberg. COVID's toll had cut down the number of barbers from sixty to below forty.

As orange dot and I enter the department, the daily prayer is being broadcast over speakers otherwise not used except when there is a fire or a tornado or active shooter. Today's prayer asks the Lord to give us strength to choose fruit and vegetables instead of junk food at snack time. The suffering caused by obesity is another of the Midwest epidemics that preceded COVID, and will—presumably—outlast it.

Ambassador remains AWOL. I'm shadowing T2 again from a distance, wearing the Kafka tiara, and hearing it all and squinting at it all and noting what I can note until, behind her back, I close the notebook. She clicks on, lost in a world of sharp talk with clinic nurses she knows well. I clip a clean piece of paper to a clipboard. With a black ultrafine-point Sharpie I draw thumbnail-sized pictures, one after the other, in straight rows, as I had planned to do at the eICU when COVID patients started expiring on screens directly to the left and right of me, ten an hour, twenty, dying alone, no relative there to mark the event with a last kiss, a squeeze of the hand. The pictures consist of riffs on spirals, triangles, squares, wing-like angles, juts of chin mouth teeth brow.

Each image is a kind of totemistic prayer that order, sense, justice, health will reign here and elsewhere. I'm thinking of the dozens of sick prisoners at the penitentiary I pass on my morning commute. Of the Cobble Hill Health Center in Brooklyn—where more than fifty residents have died of COVID. Of acquaintances recently lost. Dr. Julie Butler, age sixty-two, of Sugar Hill, Harlem. She invited us to visit her church after we moved into the neighborhood. Tom, the Galileo expert, dead in a Bronx nursing home, hours after talking to a loved one via FaceTime. I'm thinking of myself, I guess, to an extent, those parts lost forever to the jaws of my childhood house at 15 Crestwood Terrace. Ink another way of grieving. It disturbs no one, at least not immediately.

Rushing away to the Gulp Counter in the middle of the afternoon, I glimpse, through patio prison bars, a Rochester armored truck arriving at Palm Place. A guard exits the truck with an empty bag. He returns, under the overcast sky, with a full bag.

No sleep studies can now be booked in the sleep lab in Pierre, the state capital, because it has been converted to a COVID unit.

November 25
"Anybody Have a Skizzors?"

Phone dings on the commute in. It's Ivan at his security guard post at PNC bank across from Madison Square Garden. HAVE A

HAPPY WEDNESDAY! MAY THE LORD BLESS YOUR DAY WITH
PEACE OF MIND AND A HEART FULL OF HAPPINESS.

What I am blessed with when I and yellow dot report is yet
another trainer—T2 is out, why I am not told. T3, red haired
like Orientation Ambassador, puts me on notice that she usually
works from home, and instantly I understand why. She sits at T2's
desk, shaking the keyboard, yelling at the mouse, "Oh for Pete's
sake!" as her mask slips below her nose. "Either I can't remember how to type or the keyboard can't remember how to be a
keyboard!" This drama is occurring as she simultaneously battles
to adjust the desk chair to the right height. She pushes a button, the seat rises. She sits, seat sinks. Pushes button again, sits,
sinks. Nostrils expanding and expelling wet air, she stomps the
thin hard carpet with the roping boots peeking out from the bottom of her weathered jeans. Seeing this is seeing not much, but
seeing something, since this is health care during the pandemic
too, petty absurdity that not even the gravitas of COVID can kill.
I suppose that while Rome burned there were certain citizens
tinkering with their well-being similarly.

She does not bother, like previous trainers, to yell "Sugar!"
instead of "Shit!" She screams, "Shit!" This time it's because
she cannot access the catacombs of Meditech, the scheduling
system. Can't log into Voalte, the messaging system, either,
meaning no instant communication with nurses at clinic sites.
And has no access to Finesse, the phone software, and lastly fails
to breech Outlook, the email system. While observing the evolv-
ing mess, I am handed, by a long-haired lady I've never seen, a
fancy Thanksgiving card ("Welcome to the team, Ben!"). When
she moves on, I toss sequined Tom Turkey in the trash, deploy
hand sanitizer.

Bolting out into the parking lot to shove a small lunch down
my throat, I hear air rip as a National Guard jet swoops low to land
at the airport near the Crack'd Pot's pork-chop special. Hearing

it, I finally apprehend that I find no songbirds here because there are none. Vibrations from loud takeoffs and landings have made this ex-orchard inhospitable to mating, breeding, nesting. This lot is exclusively the property of birds of war: F-15s, crows, the woodpecker in my skull.

Back inside, I find T3 has not finished her lunch of French fries. She continues eating while answering phone calls. She eats by ripping down her mask below her chin, popping in a fry, yanking the mask up. Every movement is rash. When thirsty, she grabs a water bottle and drinks from it like a pirate drinking from an upside-down bottle of rum. Done sucking, her head thrashes forward in the style of a driver's-ed car-crash video, and she answers the next call, mask dangling off her neck like a bib.

I blink. The awe, the horror. Accept it! As much as they do careen, do gripe, do repeat themselves, the other schedulers, even T3 and Magical Thinker, are my new Einsteins and Aristotles and Platos and Madam Curies. The smartest people in the world to me because they know how to do the job I do not know how to do.

"Skizzors!" T3 cries next. "Anybody have a skizzors!?" It's her word for scissors. She must have a funny word, because her brain wants to outlive the boredom of knowing a job too well. She must prolong any glitch to let her intellect breathe.

Someone does have a pair of skizzors. She stands and brushes past me, panting, returns, panting, to take the next call while skizzoring paper, the paper flying.

Day ends with the irritation of a man who has to cancel his appointment because he has had a furnace problem. "Can I do the test tomorrow?" he asks. "Tomorrow is Thanksgiving," T3 snaps. "Oh," he says, as if he did not know, as if he is suffering from carbon-monoxide poisoning. She hangs up, laughing. It's another gap for capitalism to fill and fill fast. A high-priced clinic open *only* on major holidays.

December 1
New Desk

South Dakota joins short list of states (eight) where one in one thousand people have died of COVID-related causes. In Pierre, the state capital, work continues on the construction of the $462,000 security barrier around the official residence of Governor Kristi Noem, Trump Republican, who refuses to wear a mask in public.

At the eICU I had a vision of human beings tightly wrapped in sheets, hurtling through darkness toward or away from the census I maintained. Central Scheduling provokes a confused vision of worried patients in cars spattered with snot-colored winter light, speeding toward diagnostic machines that will peer into them as if they were file drawers.

On this orange-dot-day, the desk that is mine is finally mine. Amazing! Only I wore a clean white shirt and need to spend considerable time in the dust under the desk plugging in monitor cords, futzing with other hookups. I pin up my postcards. On a shelf I place a conch shell I bought on Twenty-Eighth Street in Manhattan, and a red buoy I found on the beach in Montauk, Long Island—the town where Anne and I spent our honeymoon one December. It's all supposed to make the "PTSD me" feel safer and more rooted, but after what has happened here, as I step back to view my decorating, I pity the buoy: what a disorienting spot for an Atlantic Ocean buoy to wash up! And the rest, it looks just one big slap of wind away from dispersal in a bureaucratic dust bowl. I need more alchemy! So when I craft a series of new passwords, they all include the word METS and 1986—the year my favorite team last won the World Series. When I dare to open my email box for the first time since April 17, I have 1,229 unread messages waiting to be checked, deleted, or responded to. Around that slog I continue haunting the edge of the cube belonging to T2, who again has me on her hands to educate. For the foreseeable future there can be no training in my cube because I don't have access to any of the six programs a scheduler needs to function.

T2 relates that her second job is at a homeless shelter for alcoholics in downtown Sioux Falls, a small shelter for men where the residents are allowed to have booze. She worked there last night. Thanksgiving Day she spent at the hospice where her father is dying. There are things bleaker than an ICU unit. The everyday world.

I learn there is an illness called smoldering myeloma and that a diagnosis of itching can be enough to cause a doctor to order an expensive MRI test. Thanks to a menu board near the Palm Place entrance, I discover They's soup of the day is SANTA FE.

At the Gulp Counter I quiz myself on the three kinds of echo (echocardiogram) tests: limited, complete, bubble. What is a limited echo? A memory that fades fast and does not impede your relationship with the present. Complete echo? A bully-like memory that backs you into a corner and forces you to face it. Bubble echo? A memory that floats, following you wherever you go—a depressed father whistling "Blue Skies" . . . a mother's face smudged with lipstick on her one night out a year.

December 2
To Grip a Mug

South Dakota's death toll surges past a thousand. I hear the dry cough of an unmasked employee behind me as I approach Palm Place. With haste I swipe in, pry off my tweed cap, lean toward thermal sensor as if bending to kiss a fragile seated relative but stopping short. Tenderness is what many days are missing, pandemic or not.

Between calls T2 says that she worked for the morgue at Sioux Valley Hospital for two years when she was in her thirties. I tell her that before going to work for this hospital organization I applied to be a greeter at a funeral home in Sioux Falls because I thought the hours would work with writing. Then, at the interview next to the casket showroom, was told the firm did not need a greeter but a remover—one who shows up at the hospital in a suit and wheels the dead away for embalming.

Sioux Falls, ranked the number-one small city for its business and career climate by *Forbes*.

Yellow dot and I suffer the scheduling details of a sweat chloride test. Rapunzel calls from Oncology, wishing she could let down her hair and escape work. Opal from the State Pen, she mentions clots forming in the lungs of infected prisoners. I find putting too much sanitizer on hands can make a mug very hard to grip at the Gulp Counter.

December 3
Mick Jagger Nail Polish

Frost on deflated latex snowmen and Santas that attempt to decorate the little yards in the neighborhood I drive out of. It's called Pettigrew Heights and named after one of the first two U.S. senators from South Dakota, Richard F. Pettigrew. Awnings and signs on Minnesota Avenue speak to me also. PHILIPPINE ORIENTAL FOOD STORE. SKYWAY LIQUORS. An ETHIOPIAN MARKET advertising GYROS. All collides in the urban Midwest. All comes apart.

To further bolster desk magic I pin up a pair of *London Review of Books* covers. Rural road curving by steeples of a hardy cathedral. White bird swooping toward the open door of a friendly looking white cage. Pastel islands for eyes to light on. T2 starts out training me, in her pen, but warns that since she has a meeting in the afternoon she'll be handing pink dot and me off to a new trainer, number four. I have never seen this worker wear a mask at her desk. Oh no.

Until being passed over, I do my best to remain calm and advance my scheduling education. "Clears" means a patient can have clear liquids prior to a test. A "lunger" is a lung biopsy. "Sucks Falls" is derogatory name for "Sioux Falls" in clinic nurse lingo. A FedEx employee dropped a box on his foot in the holiday rush and needs a workers' comp MRI of the foot. T2 says the workers' comp element must be cited on four different screens that flash by too quickly for me, the shadow, to absorb.

During a break I check email and learn this large health system has scheduled "Forty Days of Compassion," asking each employee to commit forty compassionate acts. But can authentic compassion, a product of the heart, be scheduled? Programmed? It's too perfect to put into fiction what happens minutes after I ask these questions. A sighing scheduler rates her last caller for the rest of the department: "Couldn't speak English! Did not understand what I was saying. Oh my god, woman!"

The first thing T4 tells me, in an oddly cheery voice, is that her brother and brother-in-law just tested positive for COVID. When I station myself nine feet behind her, in another cube entirely, she receives the message and masks up, and I thank her, inching within seven feet. Hers is yet another style of doing the job.

T4 ignores the ringing phone to talk about her Dakota life, as her hands veer and point in Mick Jagger Wembley Stadium fashion, punctuating details with sparkly purple nail polish. She is one of ten children. The town she grew up in had a population of 125 when she was growing up and now has shrunk to 30. Her grandfather lived to be 107. She has five brothers and a grown son who keeps adding to his boyhood collection of Matchbox cars and a grandson who drinks out of the dog's water dish. There's a video. Want to see it? She advises me that in scheduler slang "Jailbird" means a county jail inmate and "Pen Pal" is a prisoner at the State Penitentiary. Her other job is that of emergency room secretary. All the talk has a point. The point is to treat the affliction of Tedium.

Self-medicating with blather. With corn chips and cream cheese, potato chips and sour cream. With light beer, wine, booze. Magical Thinker on the first afternoon: "I can already taste my Ultra." Ambassador on my second morning: "I think it is a Sauvignon Blanc night." When T4 finally accepts a call, it is from an elderly woman who left her glasses in a bone-scan machine and wants them back. "Wrong number!" Click. T4 asks: "You've been trained by how many of us so far?" I tell her, adding: "At this rate I'll be the Frankenstein scheduler made up of different parts of all of you."

December 8
Shit Show

Fifty-four percent of people in the United States know someone who has died of COVID or been hospitalized because of it. Unable to handle the surge, South Dakota begins flying seriously ill patients to locations in Minnesota. During the first week of this month the state has the highest mortality rate per capita of any other state. Voice of America reports that since April there have been twenty-one suicides at the Pine Ridge Indian Reservation, 377 miles west of Sioux Falls. Tribal lands constitute over 12 percent of the state's total territory. Due to lack of health care facilities on reservations, tribal members requiring critical care—a flight nurse told me—had to be flown to Sioux Falls or Rapid City.

The world's first COVID vaccine administered outside of a clinical trial is given to ninety-year-old Margaret Keenan, wearing a Merry Christmas T-shirt, at Coventry's University Hospital in the UK. She called it the "best early birthday present."

Orange dot on badge, I learn kidney stents are not always plastic and that the gantry tilt is a way of doing a CT scan that a scheduler must remember. Menu board for They, the cafeteria, advertises fried-chicken rolls with a side of tater tots. Every facility has an IT deity and I meet the one here: Hans. But even he cannot fix nearly everything broken in this corner of Palm Place. I hear a river of whispers among schedulers I am not meant to hear but they whisper loudly when referring to my training as a "shit show. *Total shit show.*" A term I often heard flung about by eICU nurses: it means *incompetence in action.*

December 9
Where the West Comes From

Another yellow-dot shift where another call comes in from a puzzled clinic nurse who needs to make an appointment for a South Dakota patient from a town that no one has heard of—though everyone in the department but me is from the state.

Courvair. Mininden. Glory. Fredonia. Telamast. St. Jackson. I am taken with the idea that no one knows about these towns because they did not exist until recently. That west of here towns appear out of nowhere—bungalows and businesses and parking lots and streets and residents in ball caps and hoodies and denim unfurling from the windy warehouse of the spacious horizon, the biggest of the big box stores. Not one nail is struck, one slab of cement laid. Sudden towns like instant potatoes. Outsiders do not learn of their place on the map until a resident has chest pains and a medevac copter lands, or a citizen has an awful headache and requires an MRI of the brain to rule out cancer. Then health care workers spread news of the new town. This fits with another theory of mine, based on decades of day jobs, that every American, whatever their line, wherever they live, has the power to bring others news that is fantastic, addressing edges of a nation's reality heretofore unknown.

December 10
Mask Remandate

Email to pink-dotted employees from Absent Boss Barbara: "Just a friendly reminder to all schedulers to please wear your masks while working at Palm Place. I know it stinks but we have been getting some complaints that our Department has not been diligent about wearing them." I pin up a postcard portrait of Henry James (in vest) between my 9/24/20 and 10/22/20 covers of the *London Review*.

"Gnomes are really popular this year"—according to the scheduler who recently made $400 at a craft show selling them. (Yes, the craft show must go on.) There are gnomes without eyes and others with eyes. It is the department's masked consensus that gnomes with eyes are "creepy." The three weeks I've been here I've yet to hear anyone mention the disputed presidential election or the execution of George Floyd and its ramifications from coast to coast. No one mentions the vaccine. BRVMT is the abbreviation for bereavement. On 1010 WINS I hear there is a ninety-second window to get vaccine doses into the freezer after they are unpacked.

December 11
Puking in the Wastebasket

Ambassador returns on this blue-dot day, nervous as ever, popping into my cube to say she will not resume training me since she still has to complete the schedule. My training, instead, consists of thirteen different online courses required of new hires or the complete weirdness of going through such an orientation process when you have already worked for said health system for three years, seen and heard the frequent drastic disconnect between the situation on the ground and the system's professed dedication to "Dignity," "Care for the Poor and Vulnerable," "The Common Good," "Engagement," "Respect," "Justice," "Mercy," "Access to Health Care," and "The Standard of Communication." It makes me want to email one of the nun trustees and suggest we meet to discuss the writings of Thomas Merton, Gerard Manley Hopkins, and St. Augustine. None of those thinkers, if they knew what I did, would consent to the swallow test required to complete these courses by checking an AGREEMENT box. I also believe they would demand the system acknowledge a key dynamic of religion not mentioned—that moral urgency can oblige one to bypass all rules in order to do the right thing. Spirituality is no box to check. It is a complicated personal precept to live—situation by situation—and does not jibe either with the command, included here, to "like" official health-system content on social media and to report to management the name and (if possible) phone number of any Sioux Falls resident heard talking negatively about the health system.

Can public relations be substituted for honesty without there being grave damage to an institution? I am almost hopping blind by the time I finish the training, but remain able to type one sentence into an evaluation form: "I suggest this process should include a specific tutorial about the importance of respecting patients whose first language is not English. Stray negative comments about those who struggle to communicate in English have shadowed my experience working here."

Magical Thinker, in the afternoon, announces to all she is not hungry for the lasagna lunch she brought. Minutes later she is puking into her wastebasket. After being summoned into Boss Barbara's office, she again departs in tears.

December 15
Axed

The pandemic death toll in the United States surpasses 300,000 people. Yesterday morning, the first vaccine shot in the nation is given to Sandra Lindsay, director of nursing for the critical care division at Long Island Jewish Medical Center in New York City. The first South Dakota COVID Pfizer vaccinations are administered later that afternoon to Dr. Anthony Hericks and Dr. Jawad Nazir, among others, at the main campus of the hospital system I work for in Sioux Falls. Dr. Hericks says to the public: "I'm getting the vaccine to protect myself, my family, and show that this is safe. It is the right thing to do."

Early in the morning Big Boss Nadine stops at T2's cube where I am being trained. Day-job radar tells something is up. Her smile like nothing is wrong means something has happened that might be construed as wrong. Her talk strains to be casual. She describes her three outdoor holiday celebrations so far, including one hosted at a state park by her maskless son with his maskless family of Trump supporters. Her jacket still smells of smoke from the blaze they gathered around.

What has happened is this—after Orientation Ambassador completed the department's six-week schedule yesterday, her name was erased from it. She was fired. The BELIEVE sculpture no longer sits on a shelf in that cube. That shelf is bare. Photographs of her kids gone. Her cross gone and the fuzzy, blue and red Minnesota Twins blanket that had been slung across her chair. An eight-year veteran of the department, she must now scramble to find health insurance during a pandemic. While I do not know the full story, I now know why she was so nervous during many of our exchanges. Hers was the look of the "hunted employee" I first saw in the face of Harvey Katz at the New York Stock Exchange in 1987. Big soft Harvey, suit and tie flapping as he lurched into his office, slamming the door as if that noise might keep a middle manager from terminating him.

As in all the other places I have worked—Wall Street to Vermont—no coworker dares mention the name of the axed human being. Absent Boss Barbara, from wherever she is, swoops onto the scene in a cyber sense with an email announcing the date of Ugly Sweater Day.

Later, I am informed T2 will be training me the rest of the way, but can't quite believe it.

December 16
Where We Live At

The day that seven managers at a Tyson Foods pork-processing plant in Waterloo, Iowa, are fired for wagering on the number of workers at the factory who would contract COVID. In excess of 1,000 employees have contracted the virus so far. Six have died. In response, Joe Henry of Latino Forward, an advocacy group, says: "Managers don't see these people as humans. They're just part of the machinery. . . ."

I'm notified by T2 that it is time for me, clad in the yellow dot and Kafka tiara, to get more active and do the keying, as she takes calls directly behind me and gathers the data from clinic nurses that must be keyed in for each booking. This means I cannot maintain a comforting distance from her any longer. I am worried because she often snaps down her mask to drink and to eat in the cube. She does it right before we start in, and as she repositions the mask I stall, asking what she did last night, and she says that last night she worked at her other job, the homeless shelter, for six hours. A frigid night, wind chill between zero and ten degrees. One client was found in a snowbank outside. Another went to the hospital with a blood alcohol level of 4.4. "It is possible to have a lucid conversation with someone with a blood alcohol level that high—if that is where they live at," she tells me.

Then, while exchanging one-liners with nurses she knows well, she jabs her thick finger at fields I need to fill in, and the tab buttons I need to click, for otherwise I do not know what the hell to do, after a month of straight shadowing. She is as unhappy with my progress as I am: clearly dealing with much, between me and the shelter and her father dying in the hospice and her daughter, college age, living at home and engaged in distance learning. I feel more concerned for her than myself. She is at least twenty years younger than me and does not walk well, swaying when she leaves to take a call from a nurse caring for her father, a retired lineman. First procedure requested of us is "peds cardiac echo on a baby." A fitting fraught start.

The Moderna vaccine speeds toward approval. Trucks continue carrying the Pfizer vaccine into New York City as a blizzard rages there. A photograph emerges of a sister high up in the hospital hierarchy sprinkling holy water on the first box of the Pfizer vaccine to arrive in Sioux Falls.

December 17
Among Us

Air-shredding fighter jets are grounded because of the fog. During my break walk, murk blots out all but the sight of parking-lot cars, elbows of perimeter trees. The pendulous American flag next to I-90 is gone, no longer daring wind to wave it. Lunch is the crunch of a crisp late-season apple from the Cadman Plaza farmer's market in Brooklyn. Anne's mother sent us a box full of winesap apples, each wrapped in a scrap of the *Times*. Back inside, pink-dotted and cold, I splash coffee into a mug from the machine with three buttons for three choices. I choose BOLD.

Reaching T2's cube, I find a conversation in progress between schedulers. They are exchanging notes on a video game they play called Among Us. The setting, I'm told, is a space station with psycho-killer crew members aboard. I back away from the dialogue. It's a trigger. It's another position I never thought I would find myself in again, face-to-face with more smart women in the Midwest with a taste for mass murder. I flash back to my mother's three go-to slaughter stories, each—I speculate—giving a different edge of her life experience a language at last: grief a voice, rage a voice, shame a voice. One night she would tell me about Manson family women knifing pregnant Sharon Tate in California. Another night she would cite the exploits of Richard Speck, stabber of nurses in a Chicago dorm. Her last favorite was the shooting of the entire Clutter family in Kansas by Perry Smith and Dick Hickock. She giggled during the accounts as these schedulers were giggling now.

Back in front of a screen and keyboard, I am warned by T2 that I need to try harder—that whether I succeed or fail at the job is "all up to me." I can't argue with that. How would I? But more to the point is that in a Midwest that to me can seem to consist of layer after layer of dissolution due to apathy and disease and absurdity, does it matter how it is scheduled?

December 18
Mount Mansfield Stare

The blue-dotted, loudest scheduler arrives with the biggest news of the month, maybe year. Mick Jagger gestures drive it home.

She received the Pfizer vaccine this morning! "It's fine, totally fine. You sit for fifteen minutes after the shot so they can be sure you are fine. I was in and out in twenty-five minutes, including the sitting. They give you the shot in the Benedictine room in the Prairie Center. Arm of your choice." I am going to spend the rest of the day in a cube next to a cube occupied by a South Dakotan whose bloodstream has the vaccine circling in it. That is progress of a kind. Reports are that the state's first shipment consisted of approximately 7,000 doses. Shots for the rest of us are months away because we are not patient-facing employees.

I field a call from a vet who cannot recall where he was shot during the Vietnam War. I find that unspeakably sad, and during my break—standing outside the entrance to Palm Place—I call upon the steadying power of the Mount Mansfield Stare. I developed the MMS in my late twenties when I was a temporary employee in the Contracts Department at the IBM plant in Essex Junction, Vermont, at a time when the ascendant brands of Americanism were Snapple and H. Ross Perot. A few years before that, Anne and I had moved from Brooklyn to the state—like we moved from Harlem to South Dakota—seeking to stabilize costs and bolster the art pursuit. During my breaks at IBM I stood at a window offering a view of Mount Mansfield, the tallest mountain in the state at 4,395 feet. It was real. It would not, for millions of years, be reduced substantially by any force. I gazed at the gray, distant bulk like it was a light in the dark—like it was an available universe to tap, and I did feel its force of being large and unusual and hard as truth. Now I focus on the airspace above the empty lot at the end of the parking lot.

At the end of the stare I check my email on the phone, learn that retired English Professor Roald Tweet, age eighty-seven, has died of COVID. He interviewed me last summer on a radio show called Scribbles on WVIK, when I returned to my hometown for the first time in many years to give a reading at the Figge Art

Museum. "I remember you," he told me. "From when you were a kid, helping out at the Mississippi Valley Writing Conference." Arranging circles of chairs and couches for conferee gatherings, cheering up depressive poets from the Chicago suburbs, setting out sugar cookies and pouring red punch after the nightly reading. I rode my bike to the site, Augustana College, early in the morning. After cleanup was finished, I rode home in the dark, crossing a bridge over the Mississippi River on a ten-speed with the frame I had wrapped, on a whim, with flowered static paper.

Returning to T2's cube, I hear a scheduler in another cube exclaim: "I can't stand New York!" She's reacting to some item on her phone. Unspoken is the next sentence: *I love South Dakota!* I glance at T2, the one who noted South Dakota is the new New York, COVID-surge-wise. If one hates New York but loves South Dakota and South Dakota is the new New York. . . .

December 21
The Great Conjunction

Tires sliding down Ninth Street. I behold this morning's population of snowmen and Santas crumpled on lawns like mini versions of Macy's Parade balloons mowed down by bullets or COVID. I note that a year ago, around this cold time, the eICU staff participated in the Christmas Sock Exchange. I drew a number, won the goody-stuffed sock put together by a Dreamer, Estefany, the support specialist from El Salvador who entered the country when she was a small girl, swimming across the Rio Grande with the rest of her family. She had picked out a Grinch sock to stuff with American luxury items: Ghirardelli chocolate and the like. She spent more than she had to. She held, like me, the lowest-paid position in the unit. She had it down already, the special importance of generosity—its power against the selfishness and meanness that could dominate, and sour, a unit where the workers were under too much pressure.

It is the green-dot day of the Great Conjunction—when Jupiter and Mars align. It has not happened in hundreds of years. The day an official of this hospital organization, masked at a press conference, points out that in the last seven days South Dakota has once again had the highest death rate per 100,000 residents in the United States.

And it is Ugly Sweater Day, a day I shouldn't have feared. Half the department does not even wear an ugly sweater. I wear a red shirt as a way of half participating to suppress any idea that I am a total snob. The scheduler with the light-up necklace, snowflake leggings, and artificial leather sleigh sewn on the front of her red sweater with strange silver bulges on the side plus tufts of what looks like awry wiring—she does not electrocute me or force me to pose with her in a photograph or kick me with her knee-high boots. The other big participator, Magical Thinker—green-and-red sequined Styrofoam Christmas balls in her hair—does not butt brows with me either. The candy-cane pattern on her sweater does not spread like the virus to my solid-colored shirt. Boss Barbara, who suggested Ugly Sweater Day, is absent again. I suggest to T2 that ABB might have put on a sweater so ugly a force field of domestic dignity prevented her from leaving home and making a complete fool out of herself in the workplace. "Huh?" is the response.

Others type so fast I wonder if a sonic boom might occur, cubes shaking like maracas. Again I try to key appointment specifics as T2 takes the calls and I listen in. A clinic nurse addresses me directly, asking: "Why would a man want to work with a bunch of women?" Because I am on mute I can't reply. She names the last male to work at Centralized Scheduling. Though he left seven years ago, she still recalls what a bad job he did. *Don't become the next Tony*, I think, picturing an impaled Tony.

After Anne picks me up, we look for the Great Conjunction after sunset. From the driveway we spot what looks like one star but is really two.

December 29
More Whispers

Because of the blizzard, test cancellations pour in. Here's one thing I can do confidently—cancel stuff. As I repeat keystrokes, a scheduler tells how, during the last whiteout, her husband became disoriented in their rural driveway and drove into a field. She, and another scheduler who must drive a final gravel mile to reach home, will stay overnight at a motel instead of attempting a commute. Holiday gifts sent by Ambassador, before she was fired, have arrived on the porches of some of the other schedulers and they do not know what to do with them.

U.S. district judge Charles Kornmann provides the heat, writing in a decision: "South Dakota has done little, if anything, to curtail the spread of the virus. . . . [Governor Kristi Noem's] example significantly encourages South Dakotans to not wear masks. South Dakota is now a very dangerous place in which to live due to the spread of COVID-19."

I need to get out during my break regardless of the weather. Briefly free, I strip my face bare, inhaling snowy oblivion like an unmuzzled Siberian horse. I think of Joel, a few years older than me, a driver for Wheelchair Express and out in this in the 2018 Dodge Caravan. Joel wears an N95 mask, and follows the advice of Marty, the owner of the business. "In the front seats of the van turn the blower on high. In the back seats turn the blower off or put it on a lower setting, and do not circulate interior air, only bring in fresh air."

Without people like Joel and the ambulance drivers, the COVID death toll would be even higher in a state of dispersed citizens. Joel had a long career raising money for nonprofit organizations until he couldn't find work in that field any longer because, as he told me, "it's a young person's job." I met this good-natured man when we both worked for ten dollars an hour behind the front desk of the city's aquatic center.

The day ends with whispers from an orange-dotted clench of schedulers. A minute before they were trading tales of friends and relatives that had had serious COVID bouts. Lost sixty pounds. Unconscious for days. Then comes: "my cousin is a policeman, believes the conspiracies. . . ." Then: "that John Roberts. . . ." Then: "it's all connected. . . ." To keep us lying to ourselves, and disconnected. To keep us apart.

Swerving up the slushy driveway I see Anne has shoveled the walk, so I can gallop straight to my barnwood desk on the second floor and write. For months I've been dwelling on the issue of form as deadly historical events have collided and collaborated. The fragility of form. The salvation of form. The form a life takes is the form its expressions inevitably assume. The two are inseparable. And watching and/or hearing forms of humanity eroding or altogether disappearing during this plague, I have felt an urgent need to know more about what vanishes when a person (in part or fully) perishes, and when an institution falters and collapses under stress. All are products of internal and external forces—the unique result of partnerships and tensions of many sorts. Studying my particular set of essential details has led to a book-length meditation on the vagaries of form I call *The Extravagant Art of Seeing: Thoughts While Tearing Up a Novel Late One Night*. I began the work in October by ripping apart seventy-five pages of a novel draft inert for decades (but indispensable nonetheless), as if the ripping was an act of creation, the next way of composing what had long needed to be written. Then I pasted the scraps at various angles onto one hundred fifty pages of ninety pound index paper, creating a stage for annotations, the space to become a new writer again.

December 30
"What an Adventure"

Twenty-eight people in Sioux Falls are hooked to ventilators. There are—or were—just twenty-four ICU beds at our main hospital here before staff added second beds to some of the rooms to increase capacity. "Doubling up," the practice is called. Evidence that a more contagious version of the virus has spread to the United States is confirmed. A man in Colorado has come down with it. No known travel history.

It is the yellow-dot day of my first "check-in" with Absent Boss Barbara. We have hardly exchanged words since I arrived. The meeting was supposed to happen two weeks ago. After she shuts the office door her mask strap breaks. Remasked, she announces, "It'll take you nine months to learn this job at the minimum." But this does not reassure because previously I've been told six months, and anyway my training period is not supposed to last much longer than six weeks. I know what I would like to say to her: *Currently I feel as if I am doing nothing but gumming up the works of the Department.* I get out the lame: "What an adventure." And continue, babbling phrases, to stress that the next few weeks are crucial, and that to get through them I will need to improve very much, and also get the support I need from others. *That strikes the right banal but effective tone, right?*

December 31
A Party Like No Other

The last day of the strangest year could only, of course, be strange. Soon after waking, I learn more than 3,700 Americans died yesterday of COVID, then read the lead story in the *Argus Leader*: "While some plan on sleeping away 2020, others are racing for local bars for what promises to be a party like no other." Why the rush? No Sioux Falls business was forced to close. The Red Eye and the Bar Code have been open throughout. We are the land of the non-lockdown. Many businesses went to extremes to pretend America had not changed, as it was changing all around them for pandemic reasons, and they put employees at risk. No working from home. So today what really troubles Palm Place? The death of Mary Ann from the sitcom *Gilligan's Island*. Her jungle gear gone forever! Beautiful Mary Ann! It makes loss simpler to deal with, I guess, and I participate too, telling how I ran home after school to see Captain whack Gilligan with his hat as Mary Ann tittered.

They, the cafeteria, features CHEDDAR BROCCOLI BITES. The parking lot is scraped and by midmorning slicks of ice are sparkling. Between that light show, white spots of snow loom like spots on lung X-rays. T2 takes calls as I and pink dot type the names of horizon towns patients will blow in from: Tripp, South Dakota—Harabu, South Dakota. "Did you know there is such a thing as a testosterone pump?" one scheduler asks the others. An hour later I think I hear someone say: "Ishmael injections are down at ASH."

The long week is ending for the schedulers who brought bags and stayed in town for the last few days as roads were cleared. One had an unfortunate surprise last night at 3:00 a.m. that must also be talked about. Her daughter, a nurse working a night shift, called to say she wanted to move to Colorado. And this is the scheduler who dislikes not just the East Coast and the West Coast but the coast of Minnesota fifteen miles away from here, her safe zone, South Dakota. Now, though, I hear in her voice what I did not hear during her last "I hate New York" tirade. I hear a mother straining to accept a daughter's choice like a good parent—trying not to let her own prejudice interfere. Anyhow, she sighs, she can't be too damn surprised because this child loved Colorado when she visited there on a band trip when she was fourteen!

It reminds me of the eICU nurse's story about her band trip from Fargo to Louisville to perform at the Kentucky Derby. There, she told me, she saw her first openly gay person.

Other schedulers shower their exhausted colleague with sympathy. As she accepts the support, above her, on a cube shelf, rests a green and white certificate thanking her for 25 YEARS OF SERVICE—an award of paper for loyalty made of steel. She is allowed to leave early. How will she stay awake during the drive? she is asked. She will drive with the window down.

After she departs, the remaining schedulers discuss where they are going to dine on New Year's Eve . . . while also conclusively admitting they are "doing nothing" for the holiday. Tomorrow a photo will circulate of confetti falling on an ICU unit in Italy.

January 4, 2021
Periodic Unexplained Staring

Record daily number of COVID cases reported in the United States. Sandra Lindsay gets her second dose of the Pfizer vaccine. And T2 demands that I try doing it all—taking calls and keying. I don't resist. I say: "Sure, why not?" Which prompts someone to shout: "You can't scare him!" I smile. My old poker face still operational, as it has been since I was ten and scared every hour. But a poker face is of no use if you do not know how to, or care to, play poker. How little we know about one another after spending these many hours penned up together. How little we dare to convey.

A number of times, by a number of trainers, I have been warned that impatient clinic nurses are apt to hang up instead of work with a newbie. Thinking quick, I come up with a few cute lines to calm customers. The best: "Don't worry, right here at my elbow I have Linda to make sure I make no mistakes. Imagine you are talking not to Ben but to a two-headed beast by the name of Benda."

However the first call is from no nonsense "Christine at the State Pen." She wants to schedule a CT for an inmate on the mobile unit that stops by once a week. She fires off details. I hear scan of abdomen, chest, neck, fingers, toes, belt or is it chest, brain, neck, pocket. . . . I ask her to repeat. She huffs but does. I need to be pointed through the keying, every screen. Not good. The whole room is listening/judging. Panicking privately, I decide that one area I can instantly improve is my greeting. I will now say: "Thank you for calling Scheduling, Ben speaking . . ." instead of "Centralized Scheduling, Ben speaking. . . ." Any path forward is better than none at all.

At some point in the daze of this green-dot day, a clinic nurse requests an MRI of the brain with and without contrast for a child. The diagnosis is "periodic unexplained staring." I am reminded of the situation that evening when I read chapter 8 of *A Little Princess* to Anne.

> At that time it was noticed that Ermengarde was more stupid than ever, and that she looked listless and unhappy. She used to sit in the window-seat, huddled in a heap, and stare out of the window without speaking. Once Jessie, who was passing, stopped to look at her curiously.

"What are you crying for, Ermengarde?" she asked.

"I'm not crying," answered Ermengarde, in a muffled, unsteady voice.

"You are," said Jessie. "A great big tear just rolled down the bridge of your nose and dropped off at the end of it."

Sorrow we hoard—hide—puts the self at a foggy distance from the self. I know the scheduling job for me! Booking an MRI for Ermengarde, a CT for Mrs. Dalloway's consciousness, bone scan for flimsy Gatsby, and a six-minute walk for Oblomov, and on and on. Centralized scheduler for the galaxy of literary characters who have been suffering from undiagnosed ailments in some cases for centuries.

January 5
Lord Mayor TenHaken's Cure

Pinks of sunrise as news darkens. Los Angeles ambulance drivers are not transporting patients who are unlikely to live—this because of lack of hospital capacity in the region. One American is dying of COVID every thirty-three seconds. Set a watch by it.

Media reports indicate that Lord Mayor Paul TenHaken of Sioux Falls, the triathlete, who for months has dithered about a mask mandate, probably contributing to the virus spread, races to get on the vaccine bandwagon, stating that the city might spend as much as $160,000 to sell it to the public. Why one health practice promoted and not the other—not soon enough? It could be read as that American flaw of valuing innovation over reality that does not gleam, shine, sell, but *just is*. Yet something else is at work on this orange-dotted day. The fact that the state government, best at doing nothing, is not involved in vaccine distribution. Mask-resister Governor Noem has handed the job over to the two largest South Dakota health organizations, who know about the nuances of partnering with local authorities to get things done.

Magical Thinker is back at her station, feeling much better, thank you. She even tries to make me feel better after as she over-hears my (and T2's) hour-long struggle to book an MRI appoint-ment for a patient full of metal: the lower back cage, neck rods, nine heart stents, right toe implant—meaning the make, model number, year of manufacture for each device must be submitted to the MRI operator for safety reasons. "Don't worry, Benda! It'll take you a year to learn this job!" When after sixth months I was a fully functional employee at the technotangle of the eICU.

January 8
Trainer Number Five

Car aimed at Palm Place, I am thinking of the spreadsheet listing the favorite things of every department employee. One listed her hobbies as "snow globes, angels, thin blue line things."

On the way in, I see T2 is not at her desk. That means her father died at the hospice. She never takes sick days. Is never late. Needs the money, every cent. Boss Barbara awaits me, blue dot on her badge and a black eye. Another day of new things. "You'll be trained by someone else!"—trainer number five. She turns, marches into her office, fires off an email warning about dropped calls. "Limit your abandons."

T5, who manufactures eyeless gnomes in her home, enters into my cube, warning: "I am not going to say anything unless you ask me a question." Aggressively shy.

I tell her I understand how difficult (i.e., annoying) it is to train someone without having any warning, and I thank her in advance for her patience. All that is missing is the curtsey.

I get a short, high-pitched noise in response. Because I do not want anyone touching my keyboard I slyly suggest she takes calls while I key. She has no problem with that. She scoots her chair behind mine and plops her bottle of Mountain Dew on my desk, beneath the interested gaze of Henry James. She rips off the mask to drink the Dew and to eat a peanut butter brownie, her breakfast treat. In theory there is nothing wrong with any of that . . . except I'm not free to eat or drink at my own desk for fear of getting COVID from those who yank off their masks to guzzle or munch at their desks. Mine should be a SAFE ZONE. I hear her chewing thanks to the teletiara. My empathy is tested. My compassion fails to an extent, as well as my hospitality—it only follows. I am wanting to be very alone when another scheduler sticks her head into the crowded cube and shouts at T5: "You chopped your hair! It looks cute!" They talk, with me between them, too between them, for at least ten minutes and three years. Stories of car crashes are exchanged. Our visitor's daughter wrecked the family car last night. T5's daughter, the opener at Hardee's, fell asleep on the way to a shift, hit the guardrail and spun the wheel, overadjusting, and ended up in a knee-deep slough and almost drowned. "Have a good day, you two!" says our visitor, knowing we are on the precipice of a horrendous day. But horrendous is relative. I'll get better answers from T5, and more patience, if I win her trust, so I ask her about herself. I learn she lives with her second husband in Toronto, South Dakota, and has eleven grandchildren. Her favorite place to eat is the Toronto Café, where on New Year's Eve she had a flatiron steak plus a skewer of shrimp. I feel I am failing at the trust thing too until she, without being prompted, mentions the "temperature blanket" she is sewing. I don't know what that is. I inquire. This project employs a color of thread associated with the weather pattern on each day of sewing. She shows me a photo on her phone of one of these pretty blankets. Then shows me photos of the chihuahua-weenie dog mix she and her husband collect. This little breed is fond of destroying pillows. Then—further delay impossible—we try to do the work we are being paid for.

First off a nurse for the transplant team calls to arrange an X-ray, an ECHO, a six-minute walk, an EEG, and an ultrasound all on the same date, to precede a patient's afternoon appointment. We spend the rest of the morning on that single task. As I key at T5's direction, a health-system rumor floats into my mind. It dates to the eICU days. More than one nurse insisted to me that the transplant doctors, to improve their "survival statistics," kept doomed patients artificially alive until a forty-five-day survival threshold for a "successful transplant" had been met. These patients, pumped full of drugs, turned blue, brown, purple. I was shown one on a screen. These outcomes haunted ICU staff who felt they were forced to be complicit in a dubious medical practice. One nurse railed: "Some of those transplant patients look like they've been dug up at the graveyard and brought to the hospital."

After lunch T5 and I book a string of simpler appointments, before pausing again to give our nerves a rest. Mentioning an upcoming October trip to a NASCAR event in Myrtle Beach, South Carolina—a trip that would introduce her to the ocean for the first time—T5 admits: "Really, I've never seen anything fascinating in my life. I would like to travel. Go to Niagara Falls. The Grand Canyon."

I carry the heavy comment home. Never a trip out of the Midwest, to a place able to shock her. Does it speak to her lacking the imagination to be fascinated by eccentric South Dakota? Or of an imagination that never found its match here, not even in gnomes?

January 11
The Little Tramp

The day Anne's parents on Schermerhorn Street in Brooklyn are eligible to receive the vaccine. The day I go to work and find there is no one to train me because T2 is absent due to her father's demise, and T5 is working from her home of crafts. "Leave," commands Boss Barbara. "Tomorrow. . . ." A sixth person will train me. I depart a bit stunned. I showed up to my job twenty minutes ago, and I am not at my job. It makes no sense. I don't have a car parked outside because Anne had errands to do and dropped me off. For the first time since the first day, I wander into They, the cafeteria. It is empty. I sit. As I collect myself I hear footsteps that get closer, closer: it's an unmasked employee and frozen bagel headed toward a toaster I've accidently sat right in front of. Dear god! Out I go. It's a beautiful day, the sun bright, the temperature mild. I make a sudden decision to walk home, take control of my destiny. Walking usually is a key to equilibrium for me. I'm happy at first to see no one else on the industrial park streets, ultimately socially distanced, *breathe deep Charlie Chaplin you are on your way again.* A half mile into the tramp I hear fifing of a killdeer! The first I've heard since April! I smell the sharp scent of freshly cut lumber. Smooth blue roux of the sky above. La-di-da. Only that woodpecker in my skull starts in, and a feeling of disorientation grows. Did our house burn down with Anne in it? I imagine fire flicking out broken windows. I'm unable to get to her to help! I feel absolutely alone out here as I did when I was fourteen, showing the world my skeletal angles during the anorexic bout and seeing a world not seeing me, not wanting to see. How will we get back to New York City? Our friends? Anne's parents? I'm on the wrong side of the canal dividing the district. Can't find a place to cross over. Keep fucking running out of sidewalk as semitrucks thunder by, forcing me to crisscross the desert of FOR RENT warehouses tank fabricators data shredders Dakota Splash Ice Supply cabinet factory . . . until I end up on a vacant road leading directly to the gothic turrets of the State Penitentiary, and stop right there. I dial Anne, quite upset with the health system but more upset with myself. I believed it was a nice day for a walk. Days are not nice now.

January 12
Clear View Lady

Trainer 6 has been with this hospital organization for forty-one years. She is one of those who were whispering about conspiracy theories at the end of a recent shift, but I press that aside, listen. She started out as ward secretary when appointments were kept in one big book. No labyrinth of pea-green screens to click through through through. No reams of data about appointments to log. Patient name is all, and test time. There was only one CT machine in the city back then. She uses phrases like "Excuse my French" and "This doctor writes like a chicken" (referring to a faxed written order).

Her husband was the South Dakotan who got lost in his own driveway. She went to a one-room schoolhouse in the 1960s. She lives in the country because she is a "clear view" lady—doesn't like small towns cluttering the landscape, let alone cities.

T6 shows me her "go-to" binder containing info about the hundreds of procedures that might be requested by a clinic caller. The binder is a photo album with plastic sleeves populated with cards. She tells me I should have a reference just like it, although she does not take into account that it took her twenty years to build this one, and no one mentioned that I should create such a book until this moment.

Hearing the news, I feel my first twinge of absolute hopelessness during a shift. I try to jolly myself out of it by speculating that at home T6 has an identical book filled with photographs of exactly the way she likes her eggs done, toast done, steak done . . . a tome of tastes she brings to restaurants and insists be shown to the cooks. These six trainers have unveiled six different ways of doing the same job. The ways cancel each other out. Orange dot over yellow dot over pink dot over blue dot over. . . .

T6 isn't sure about getting the vaccine, she says, after we book an MRI for an eighteen-year-old who just got a shot and now is having "word-find difficulty" and seizure-like activity and twitchy eyes and headaches. Clear View Lady isn't sure about the vaccine at all, though she knows these symptoms could have nothing to do with the vax.

January 13
Double Duty

President Trump impeached for a second time by the House of Representatives. The Javits Center in Manhattan opens as a vaccine distribution center after serving for months as a field hospital. Seven days running the United States has broken its daily death total record. More than 380,000 Americans have perished of COVID-19.

For the first time I am handling the phones *and* the computer keying. T6 and I are sitting in my cube. As we are getting settled, she states she believes the virus was purposely released by China in order to ruin the president and adds she does not watch the news anymore: too depressing. She points at my postcard of the arched tile ceiling of the Grand Central Oyster Bar. I tell her that is where Anne and I had our first date in 1987. She nods. She shakes her head, unable to resist saying she could never live in New York City, being a "clear view lady." I am unable to resist asking if she has ever visited the Royal Bake Shop in Centerville, thirty miles from here. She has. It is an old-time screen-door bakery famous for its Zebra Donut consisting of "marbled vanilla and chocolate dough, fried, glazed, and dunked in chocolate frosting." The place was family owned for many decades before being sold to a middle-aged employee who had started working there when he was in high school. There are antique glass cases of baked goods, a wooden floor, and the original string dispenser. I explain to T6 that what I love most about New York City is shopping at little neighborhood stores and specialty shops just as friendly as the Royal Bake Shop. On Court Street in Brooklyn. On Ninth Avenue in Manhattan. Getting to know the counter help and even the owners—learning from them how to cook shad roe or venison tenderloin or soft-shell crabs or calves' liver. Esposito's butcher shop. Caputo Bakery. Lobster Place. "There are still many little stores in New York City, stores you can't get lost in." She's done nothing to convince me there is a virus conspiracy—have I taught her anything about New York City? I cannot tell.

Kafka tiara rings. The nurse asks if I've gotten the five automated orders and one written order per a set of diagnostic tests to be booked "pronto." Quick I check the fax queue dwelling in a folder within a folder within a folder. I find the faxes, which then need to be coded individually and copied to other folders, before the booking task can be initiated. The job, despite my being helped, takes three hours.

In the afternoon, without warning, frustrated with glitches in a software program we are using, my trainer makes a claw of her hand and squeezes my shoulder hard. The sudden touch of an older adult. That is a trigger. She doesn't mean to do harm, I know. She meant it as a friendly gesture of solidarity, I know.

That night I dream of the night during my urban Iowa child-hood when a babysitter's stoned boyfriend grabbed my shoulders hard, lifted me and spun me around over his head, and tossed me out the door onto the snow-covered front porch. A blizzard was in progress. I was wearing pajamas and socks. I did not cry out for help as I climbed to my feet, the oldest of six trying to be a solid anchor for the younger ones while mother and father were at a movie at the Capital Theater. I walked to the front door, shaking off snow. I found the door locked. I knocked, heard laughing inside. I did not cry then either. I put my head down. I shuffled through side-yard drifts to the back door, staying close to the wall, remembering the stories of pioneers who froze to death steps from their cabins. I found the back door locked. Babysitter and boyfriend stood in the kitchen window, taunting. She was a member of my Aunt Carolee's church. She slapping boyfriend for being such an enjoyable maniac in overalls. I sat then on the snowy stoop steps. My teeth were chattering. I would not die like the Little Match Girl, I had no matches to strike. I waited for the adults to finish playing games and let me in. There are those who run from nightmares and those who search for new ways into the nightmare from which they have been ejected, especially if they think—or have been taught—that that is all they have.

January 14
The Clock Strikes Twelve

Last day working with T6 is the most nerve-racking. I need to be ready to pull away if she tries "the claw" move again. I'm too anx-ious to deliver the cheerful phone retorts I keep inventing to make my position stronger: "Beware! You're talking to NKOB or New Kid on the Block." "You're not going to benefit from the usual artistry here, so in advance I thank you for your forbearance." To be said after an error: "Shoot . . . sorry, shoot . . . hey, you'd think I was in a Hollywood western." "Not Dan, the name is Ben, Ben just like the big bell in London."

Mailboxes are removed from some street corners in South Dakota to prevent extremists from placing bombs in them.

January 18–19
Elephant Rabbit

United States surpasses 400,000 COVID fatalities. T5 and I bumble through bookings. Email notification that a clinic nurse with nineteen years of experience died yesterday in the ICU of COVID, and another email regarding the eternal mask problem: "Disposable masks are now to be replaced half way through a shift instead of being used for the entire shift. N95 mask reprocessing will be decreased from 5 disinfection cycles to 2 because . . . some studies have shown that it is possible that an N95 mask protects less the more it is worn." It took the hospital seven months of the pandemic to discover this. When I get home I do not lock three doors behind me as I did during the summer. It's not that I feel safer. I believe less in the ability of locks to protect.

The inauguration of Joe Biden and Kamala Harris—the retreat of disgraced president Trump to Florida. Out the kitchen window, as specifics of the ceremony seep from a radio, I see a rabbit I have not seen in a long time, the rabbit that Anne and I call "Elephant Rabbit." Shope papilloma virus has caused a trunk-like growth on the rabbit's head that is inches long and dark and wobbly and cumbersome, covering one eye. I watch the creature's effort to eat, how it tilts the deformed head sideways to allow mouth access to the feed we've scattered, and after eating retreats to the edge of the house where it is warmer, and naps, good eye shut.

January 21
Posturography

The entrance temperature scanner claims I have a temperature of eighty-four degrees, meaning I am dead. I step back. I try again to earn my pink dot. Same result. Is this what dying in your sleep is like? You go to work anyway, the freed soul of the rat still seeking the wheel? My shoulder is tapped. I'm told to remove eye frames. The machine is registering the temperature of plastic, not the temperature of skin.

Another Boss Barbara "check in" occurs in the office, where she tells me that she listens to music while typing. How civilized. I don't want to appear totally negative, while feeling totally negative. I tell her: "I'm trying to get comfortable with being very uncomfortable." She responds: "Your calls will be recorded and rated for efficiency."

I resume training with T2 in my cube. Wearing the same gray hoodie as always, she sits to my left. Her father is buried. She yawns. To my right sits a new binder containing my notes from the past two months. I have recopied many of them, and placed test details in alpha order: cisternogram, discogram, posturography. . . .

Over the top of the next cube the flash of nail polish, the Mick Jagger hands and the face that goes with. T2 is asked about the funeral and she tells a tale of pants. Owning only jeans, she was forced to buy pants to wear to the event, which irked her. The cost bothered her so much that after she got home from Penney's she went through her closet again to look for a pair of pants she vaguely recalled purchasing years ago. I imagine her in the closet digging. What went through her mind as she dug? Was it really about money to be saved? Or her father? Or both? An homage to a penny-pinching man? Or the need for a distraction, to get in there in the shadows, and away from the starkness of death filling the home? She looked long enough, she tells everyone, and hard enough, despite all else needing to be done, that she did find the old pants, and returned the new pair for a refund. "I'm cheap," she says.

Chekhov, South Dakota. It's out of that well of literature about ordinary people and the extraordinary things they do to get by.

At last I place my phone on READY and it rings. Recorded, I think. Efficiency, I think. "Need a PFT with ABGs," snaps a clinic nurse. I blank out. I falter. After pissed off T2 takes charge and books the appointment, I am told: "You looked like a deer in headlights." I say nothing. My mouth is stuck under the two masks. I cannot form a word for more than a minute as she asks again and again: "How. Could you. Have handled that. Better?"

January 22
"I Need Help!"

I return to Palm Place, power of speech restored, blue dot applied. I request a few hours to go over my binder. This is allowed after a conference between Boss Barbara and T2. Mercy? Pity? I don't care. I'm just happy not to answer phones.

As I sit, quizzing myself about loop recorder removal, a scream comes from across the aisle. Magical Thinker. "That bitch! She was so rude to me! She had no right to be so rude to me!" She is crying. "Someone please help me with this ultra-sound! I don't know what to do! I need help!" No one comes to her rescue. She's not asking in the proper fashion. No one wants to catch her panic. Then, slowly, after more than fifteen minutes, she is visited by various colleagues, who attempt to console her, not effectively.

The incident points out something I need to understand. Because of the number of different tests that are scheduled, it is not uncommon for even the most senior schedulers to ask one another for aid. It's expected I will do the same when I go solo . . . but nothing about asking for help in the Midwest is easy for me. Each request is accompanied by a terror that help won't be there—as it was not before, when I was ten and twelve and fourteen. Without achieving independence here very soon I could not say how it would end.

January 25
Solo

Approaching the Palm Place entrance, I am thinking of words Anne left me with: "Just try and bob on the surface, go with the flow." She watches from the car. I turn once. We exchange a wave. I enter, lean, am told I am not feverish, apply green dot, swab steamed-up lenses, and note an interesting chalked misspelling on the cafeteria menu board. Soup of the Day: CHESSY POTATO.

When I open my email box I find a message notifying the group: "This is Ben's first day alone on the phone. Help him if he asks for help." Does this happen to young nurses? Are they suddenly thrust onto the front lines to care for patients, without any warning, after conveying they do not feel they are ready to deliver good care?

Surprise is the environmental element that PTSD works least well with. Once I click READY, I know I'm one call away from the day being smashed into smithereens by a call I can't handle. I've got to have another plan today other than answering calls. It's the obvious plan, a survival plan. *Duck calls* rather than make mistakes that could waste valuable hospital resources and inconvenience patients, or even endanger their health. Booking a test with contrast dye for a patient with an allergy to dye could easily happen if I get flustered. I duck calls by keeping my phone status on WORK instead of READY. I duck calls by going to the bathroom and staying there.

The first call I dare to take proves the strategy is justified. It is a call from a nurse who needs to schedule an emergency MRI for a child whose leg was shattered over the weekend and has developed, the doctor thinks, an aneurysmal cyst. "We need an MRI with and without contrast on left humerus this morning!" I stand up. I request help. The other schedulers are busy typing and talking. They stay busy. I have to tell the nurse I will call back. By the time I get the information I need and do call her, she informs me "other arrangements" have been made. She does not explain. What I know is that a child needed help, a boy, and I could not help because help that had been promised to me did not materialize. Another wicked circle is indeed complete.

When I dare to click READY again, a clinician asks for a test for a condition I have to ask her to spell. She blurts "basically it is to place a drain in an armpit." What? Help!

T3 cuts short an in-progress story about her dog-water-drinking grandson's possible COVID infection to dash to my side, mask far below her nose. Jagger hands pointing, she talks me through a HIDA scan booking that involves a secondary appointment for gastric emptying, a test that is only done at 7:00 a.m. and 11:00 a.m. at the main hospital. An hour later, when I am READY again for trouble, it's a call from a clinician who needs to schedule the removal of a port that was placed in New York City in a patient who recently moved to Sioux Falls. Never done that. Help!

I learn something could be worse than the first day at Centralized Scheduling, or any other shift I have ever worked. Yes, this is the most unpleasant and chaotic day in three decades of working with data in settings where accuracy is the priority and deadlines matter. More chaotic than the NYSE crash in October of '87 or the night before Christmas at Macy's Santaland or my last eICU shift: screens filled with asphyxiating workers from the

Smithfield meat-processing plant and a COVID-exposed nurse five feet behind my back, clicking a keyboard and yawning. Not once does Boss Barbara check in with me. Afraid to, most likely. Afraid of being confronted with news that does not fit with her concept that I am ready to go.

Of twenty calls I could not manage to dodge or duck, I needed prolonged assistance with thirteen, meaning another employee rushing to my side, partially masked, breathing hard, our faces less than a foot apart for fifteen minutes, forty minutes, an hour . . . the specter of COVID making it extra difficult to pay attention. At the end, when an oncology nurse faxes two orders, one for labs and a CT on a Thursday, and the other for an MRI on a Tuesday, both of these appointments for the same patient, and requiring the booking of a "live" (as opposed to "dead") translator in each instance, I don't cry out for help, I whimper and slump in my swivel chair.

T3 hears and clomps over in her boots. She slurs her words. Is she drunk? First she has her elbows on my desk, tail high in the air. Then she strangely kneels on the floor beside me rather than sitting on a chair. Breath courses out of her mouth as she says, "What is it? What in the name of alfalfa is it? Come on, what?" "I . . . I'm fatigued . . . I don't even know where to start." "Okay, here. . . ." One ability does kick in then, that talent for disassociation: I recall she likes the frozen garlic-butter mussels from Costco as she looks at orders and tells me the freaking tabs to hit, what freaking words to type. She speaks in the scheduler trance tone as if details mean nothing, as if they are not even words. The last thing I do at her direction is book an interpreter for each appointment, and then, alone again in my cube, I stare up at Henry James, mutter: "That last call took minutes off my life."

It's for him, just him, but someone else hears, the second-newest scheduler. She wants to help me now. She helps by telling me about her heart attack over the summer. Her fiancé did CPR on her and saved her life. She's a decade younger than me.

I had thought her the fittest member in the department until this moment. Athletic build. Running shoes actually used for running. She laughs, adding, "It might have been the job stress." I grab backpack. T3 bellows at my back: "Shee you tomorrow, Ben!"

January 26
Funayama Lithograph

Wake up, planning on going to work—to give the job one more shot. But shortly after rising, I think of the Japanese lithograph that hung on the wall of Funayama, our favorite sushi place on Greenwich Avenue in New York City, just off Sixth Avenue. It depicted the foamy lip of a tidal wave poised above a sedate seaside village that in a second or two will no longer be there. My eyes moisten as I picture that picture, and then tears tickle again. Anne hears. She steps into the upstairs hallway, outside our bedroom, and murmurs: "If you can't go back, you can't go back."

As soon as I can that day I email Boss Barbara explaining I had hoped the hodgepodge approach to orientation involving six different trainers would amount to having wings to fly on my own, but that "instead of two wings, or even one, it felt like I had six stray feathers stuck into random places, and none of them able to flap." Her response does not include a suggestion of more training. It starts: "I will need to know by tomorrow morning if you wish to keep your employment or not. If you do, today will have to be counted as an unscheduled absence." It ends: "the job was going to be a baptism by fire because with a job like this there is no other way." Had "fire" been mentioned in my interview, I never would have taken the position.

Lower-level employees who are not unionized often do not feel they have options when threatened with dismissal in a nation servitude has built from start to finish. But since I have been diagnosed with a disability, and noted this on my application, the inopportune use of the phrase "baptism by fire" to refer to the culmination of the training process allows me immediately to seek support from the head of Human Resources. Without hesitation she agrees I deserve an orderly work environment, devoid of flames, as I continue to heal. She understands the greatest determiner in the success of a hospital employee is the quality of the orientation process preparing them for the intense and unusual situations common in health care. And she knows the leader of any hospital unit or department, if their authority is to be legitimate, must be able not only to *command* but also to *express* plans and expectations in a range of ways. The catch? I have only four weeks to find a new position with her aid.

January 27
The Lure Thirty-Two Stories in the Sky

Anne and I execute a plan to evacuate lucky charms from Palm Place. We arrive at 6:00 p.m., half an hour before the facility automatically locks, and an hour after the Scheduling Department closes. There should be no one there. Of course it is possible someone will be there. I have a mundane retort at the ready: "Easy come, easy go."

At 6:02 p.m. I swipe in, lenses steamy, double masked. No one is in the department. Not T1–T6. Not Magical Thinker or Absent Boss Barbara or Big Boss Nadine. I strip the bulletin board of the Charles River, the Grand Central Oyster Bar, Henry James. I decide to leave the two *LRB* covers behind as succor for my successor. I grab the bud vase, the conch shell, the Montauk buoy, the unopened boxes of tea I could not drink, tea being for sipping, not gulping at a counter. Walking away, I think of the memorable temporary worker who one summer surfaced at Facts On File, the reference publisher where I worked for twenty years. He could have been an actor like Chet, who traveled with Theodore Bikel in a production of *Fiddler on the Roof* between stints as a salesman of Facts On File products. Or he could have been a writer like me. Or a dancer. Or a musician. His was a brief assignment, but he did not leave his cube bare— he decorated it with a blown-glass globe the size of a baseball with a trout fly suspended inside, vivid tufts of blue, orange, red threaded to the hook. I found it difficult to pass his cube on my way to the copy room. The trout fly looked like the act of casting, usually all air, confined in an airless space. The artifact of angling dangled right over his head while also pointing out how far he was from any trout stream—a lure thirty-two stories in the sky!

But I had learned enough at Palm Place to catch up— finally—to the full meaning of his gesture. The globe reflected cold fluorescent light—turned it to living sparks. The loveliness of resilience was reflected there. Sometimes survival of the heart, spirit, and mind—those fonts of art—means quietly sticking it out—nesting wherever you have landed in need of a paycheck. Sometimes survival means fighting bosses; sometimes it even means running from an institutional disaster too big for an individual, without real power in the organization, to address adequately. That temporary telemarketer in short sleeves cared enough to bring the permanent passion for fishing with him wherever he worked, punching buttons, for a week. Passing that globe was a brush with fearlessness that an identity, even when fragile and marginalized, can project. I had been afraid for his dream. He wasn't afraid. *Making the next blank place dear, and the next, is lending a life a permanent where.* When I emerge Anne waves from the car. A minute later, we roll away.

LOG 3

Reckoning at the Prairie Center

February 2021
"Well, What Are Your Ideas?"

If I did not—as a writer trying to cover living expenses—belong in a support position in a telehealth ICU with its soundtrack of suffocating Americans during a pandemic, the short-lived transfer from there to Central Scheduling taught I was a worse fit in a department dedicated to the robotic art of booking as many pricey procedures as fast as possible to keep the hospital system solvent. Had I been thinking more clearly before snapping up the job, I could have drawn guidance from my only other clerkish day job with a health care connection prior to 2017.

At an Electronic Data Systems facility on the edge of Burlington, Vermont, I joined other Kelly temps assigned to reject or accept Medicaid claims according to rules we had not been properly taught. The nauseating notion that I might accidentally deny a legitimate claim inspired me to approve every single claim—tap Y, tap Y—despite dread that I might at any moment be tapped on the shoulder, caught. Turned out only speed mattered there also. Boss Quail, always going to, or coming from, a meeting, sang my praises: "Boy you're fast!" But I despised the charade.

Where would my next perch be, if any? First I must pass an in-person screening by the head of HR prior to our attempt to locate a third, more suitable, hospital position.

I enter the building called Plaza 4 on the main medical campus wearing a light-blue dress shirt under a peacoat and the rigid, affable expression of one trying to look relaxed when not. Will I be articulate? Will I present well?

I pick up the wall phone, introduce myself. Receptionist buzzes me in. The small humorless waiting room could make anyone wonder: *What next?*

"Ben?"

Masked HR head. I greet her. We enter the room where nurse Patrice waits in scrubs. She is a member of the National Guard just back from a stint of service. Her specialty is witnessing meetings that have ADA implications, as my case did, given the letter on file detailing the PTSD diagnosis. I strip off the blue coat, revealing an unwrinkled button-down. I arrange coat over a chair and take my seat at the broad conference table with the glowering brown surface.

We briefly hash over the Central Scheduling debacle.

"Barbara told me three people trained you."

"There were six. I'll never forget them. I can supply the names."

"No, that's alright. Well, what are your ideas? Full-time? Part-time? PRN?"

PRN status meant no benefits, but when the chief benefit for a twenty-four-hour part-time employee involves paying more than $600 monthly for health care (for two people) the wonder of the word *benefits* wilted.

"Part-time, no more than twenty-three hours. Or PRN."

"What about being a valet?"

"I'm sorry. A rental-car key fob can send me into a tizzy."

They gawk, having never, I think, heard a man admit vehicular ignorance.

"Well, *what are* your ideas?'"

I glance down at the clipboard to be sure I stay on message.

"A calm and orderly environment. A job I can grasp quickly, in a few days. One that will take advantage of my skill set: congeniality, reliability, accuracy."

"Okay, you search hospital job listings and we will too. Let's talk on the phone in a week about what we've found. We'll set up the interviews for you."

I have passed the smell test. I stand. They stand. Goodbye.

The first call does not go well. It is clear that these helpers, while saying some of the right things, wished to redeposit me ASAP anywhere and be done with the problem. I reject their idea that I join the army of inquisitors whose only task is to screen visitors for COVID. The jobs were listed as temporary, lasting six months. They next suggest secretarial openings in Plastics and Pain Services. I'd looked into those options but each required a familiarity with complex billing software I had never used. After the call ends, my concern about "our four-week process" is such that I apply for a cashier's job at the Sioux Falls Food Co-op, but do not get a call back.

The next week the duo recommends the role of Supply Chain Technician, another name for lifter of heavy boxes of medical equipment in a warehouse. When I demur, citing bad knees, they request proof, which my acupuncturist supplies.

The third week it is suggested I might draw blood at clinics.

Jesus, stab people for a living? "I thought you had to go to school to do that."

"They can train you in a week."

"Just a week! To be honest, I'm squeamish. . . ."

On February 22 the U.S. COVID death toll surpasses a half million. As the end of the short month nears, I have the trauma specialist I am working with send another letter to HR, explaining the need for just the right job, and it wins me enough time to spot a listing for a sixteen-hour-a-week concierge position in a side lobby of the Prairie Center, a newer campus building surrounded by landscaping that vaguely references native shrubs.

I interview via Webex. I get hired. Again I am earning under $15 an hour, but funds remained from the 401K I had cashed in last year, and there is a damn convincing argument to make for rejoining the system in the first tolerable capacity found. What safer option did I have? Few workplaces other than hospitals require masks in the city now.

Besides, the notion of reporting to a cozy lobby on the edge of it all—serving a day-surgery unit—had promise. No computer work. No phone pressure. Colorful day-job shirts I'd collected over many years could be worn without hesitation. The locale guaranteed a nearness to sunlight and other outer realities previous jobs were perilously disconnected from. It was pure human relations: talk functioning as the choral creation of a day, person by person. The doorman faced outward.

And for the first time at any little job I'd have a kind of underling—the temp-taking screen on a stalk. He'd handle the techno-Kafka tasks! I named him Ernie Temerity because he never stopped saying, "Success . . . Success . . ." to arriving staff who were still watching COVID casualties climb.

March 26
Patient Facing

For the first time since January, South Dakota logs more than one thousand new COVID cases, and is designated a "hot spot" in the latest White House report.

For the only time, I am spared the usual clock in of 4:30 a.m. I roll off to the sole day of training at 8:00 a.m. A confident Cliff Avenue digital billboard tells me: YOU ARE NEEDED. And in the next cycle: YOU HAVE VALUE.

As instructed, I park in the South Lot. I walk toward the Prairie Center sipping air through two masks, cloth and surgical. It is sunny. I hear birds. Warmest spring in years. I am scheduled to receive my first dose of the Pfizer vaccine in nine days.

Name aside, the complex reminds me of a mini version of Manhattan's Winter Garden, which faces the Hudson River and absorbs light like a crystal sponge. Dr. Forge, the acupuncturist who sent HR the Knee Letter, practices in a first-floor office at one end of the atrium, near the baby-grand piano visited often by a volunteer who plays wobbling chords of Queen's "Bohemian Rhapsody." There is a shop selling aromatherapies in vials and wooden syllables of inspiration: BELIEVE, LOVE, HOPE. The Quarry, a cafeteria featuring a wood-burning pizza oven. Benches. High tables and stools. Berms of plantings. Two faux waterfalls with recirculating currents. Rost Meditation Room, named for a late director of anesthesia and nestled behind a molded facade designed to reference ancient eroded granite spires called the Needles that attract tourists to Custer State Park far to the west. Towering atrium panes are etched with images of prairie grass more resembling shredded dot-matrix printouts waving in wind. The faint gurgle of water commingles with the hum of the HVAC system and intercom announcements. Patients from five states

(Iowa, Nebraska, Minnesota, South Dakota, North Dakota) are served by the facility.

The lobby of the day-surgery unit is on the opposite end of the atrium from the "Bohemian Rhapsody." Movement-triggered whoosh of a sliding door to a foyer populated with a few wheelchairs. Whoosh of a second door.

"Are you Ben?" my new trainer asks, an angular person in a pantsuit standing next to a considerable desk starring a shapely lamp.

"Glad to meet you," I say.

"I'm Jolene." She was the Super Concierge, I had been advised.

The place has the feel of a discreet lobby of a boutique hotel. Upholstered brown chairs against a wall. On one side of the chairs is the staff entrance for Radiation Oncology. On the other side of the chairs is a table stocked with masks and a carton of latex gloves. Next to that stands Ernie the screen and—who else?—Ernie Jr., the hand-sanitizer stalk. The two elevators stop on two floors, the surgery unit and the inpatient rehab unit. A glass door leads to the atrium's fantasia. Jolene has been the concierge here for six years, ever since figuring out she despised retirement.

For the next four hours I observe earnest Jolene and take too many notes and feast on the view of sun flashing on lot windshields. It's as if burning chariots are parked in rows, not Fords and Hondas. When I look down I see, under the desk, a large cardboard box containing dozens of smaller boxes full of masks. A literal fortune in protection! For kids there are petite masks bearing images of Donald Duck.

Employees bow to Ernie, are blessed, apply the day's color of screening dot to photo-ID badges. Between twenty and forty surgery patients enter the lobby "on a daily basis." Children having tonsils out or ear tubes inserted. Adults in for colonoscopies, gallbladder removal, mastectomies, hernias, dental work. After the patient and their companions are screened, the concierge applies wristbands that match the color of the day's employee-badge dot. "If a patient flunks the temp test call upstairs." A nurse comes down, takes it from there. "If a patient requests parking help, page the valets at the main entrance." One of the ruddy men in green jackets will hurry over and park the RAM truck.

Through the lobby shuffle cancer patients holding hands with loved ones. They are heading toward treatments delivered elsewhere in the Prairie Center. In charges a patient in the wrong place: "Google Maps says this is Plaza 3!" There are actual maps to give these mistaken souls when they settle down. Each shift I'll have a list of the patients scheduled for this surgical center, and a list of the patients being treated at the main OR, on a meandering campus that has accreted over many blustery Dakota decades, guided by no coherent master plan. You are only as good as the lists they provided you with in jobs like this—lists you did not produce. An accurate list sets you up for a good day. A flawed list, the opposite.

Vaccine angst is an early recurring theme. A middle-aged man who has had the shot tells of his wife who refuses the jab, and a son, a teacher, who won't get it. He shakes his head, boards the elevator. Jolene tells me about her two Pfizer shots, and of the pandemic's start here. In March 2020 she was informed one Friday that she was to start screening patients for fevers starting on Monday. "Will I be given a mask?" she asked. No, she was told. High-level administrators feared it might frighten patients. Over the weekend anxiety mounted. Finally, after attending church, she called her son, a doctor. He told her not to report—"Blame it on me." The leave lasted until recently. Her supervisor (now mine) respected the decision.

Jolene slipped her fate out of the institution's grip at exactly the right time. That was the dance for any worker to master—knowing when to obey and when to evade. As one who had been in a tower in Manhattan on the morning of September 11, 2001, the attack had introduced a question that never could be answered. If a plane hit my building, and the intercoms ordered me to shelter in place, would I have? Or would I have rushed down the stairs? The followers of directions died that day.

The closing-down task Jolene stresses is the unplugging of the lamp, and wrapping of the cord around the stem, once, twice, three times. . . . It looks to me like she is trying to lasso light to bring home with her. She keeps wrapping as I avert my eyes.

March 29
Birth of Chirp

Arrive at 4:30 a.m. and, from my lobby perch, observe phases of sky from predawn to dawn. The dark of a thicket melds into an aqueous black that turns coal blue, paler blue, until the sun is out and adding its white and yellow to the conversation.

I start developing my lobby script. Birds are born knowing their songs and where to sing them. Humans must again and again discover their songs, locate the venues for them.

Ernie is Ernie to me but to visitors and patients he will be a "gizmo"—nonbureaucratic word, fun slang to sling and to hear, potentially puncturing the tension when a COVID doubter parades in. "If you would, step in front of that gizmo. . . ."

Before "good morning," I add, "Hello folks," and after it, "My name is Ben." The best part though is yet to come: "Now I'm going to send you up to the fourth floor. That is the surgery unit itself. Deep breath. First part is done. You're right where you need to be. When you step out of the elevator, look to the left and you'll see a registration area about fifteen feet away. Go over there and someone will start taking care of you."

Patient with an emotional-support poodle strapped to chest tells me her name, and the dog's name. I find her name on the list. Masked atrium window washers enter the lobby seeking a restroom. It's like seeing a Ziegfeld line-dance of jangling tool belts and boots when they go the way I point.

During the first week of a new position, you do things you never do again. Today, as the temp nears seventy, I take an unrelaxing break stroll around the bubbling brown water of the faux waterfall outside the Prairie Center, facing Cliff Avenue.

March 30
MA in Dot Management

Overnight there has been a terrific wind. Gusts in our downtown neighborhood sounded like volleys of artillery. The event pushed the charnel smell of the Smithfield slaughterhouse out of the city and heralded a drastic temperature drop. Today the high is thirty-six. Vermont's weather was as extreme but not nearly as dynamic. Here you can experience three different extreme weathers in a single day. Arriving in the lobby, I plug in the lamp with its glow diffused by grayish crushed crystal.

Then I go about one of the funniest tasks I've been asked to do at any day job. Meticulous Jolene does it, insisting I do it too. I peel the day's hue (green) of employee badge dots off the spool, embroidering the edge of the table offering free surgical masks to those without them. It's like punctuating the lobby with Day-Glo ellipses. It's an effort to save employees the effort of peeling off the dots. What service! How will the staff use these split seconds we are saving them? Will they ever amount to ten minutes of extra leisure? I can't resist poking fun at the protocol. I tell entering staff: "I have a Master's degree in Dot Management from Purdue."

I'm already growing so used to the sliding-door soundtrack of airy abrasion I hardly hear it. Security lights reveal nurses approaching the lobby entrance before sunrise. They lug Crock-Pots for potlucks and shift bags. Every posture is a personality's outline, every gait a signature—bouncy, scooting, beeline, limping. Some have been with this system for ten, twenty, thirty or more years. I really do not know any of them yet, but I try to say "Good morning" with equal energy to all. We share a commitment to work, an understanding of illness.

With hospital COVID restrictions loosening a bit, red-vest volunteers are returning systemwide to enhance the patient-care experience and assist units in small but important ways. They give directions. They push wheelchairs. A different volunteer clocks in every day to help in the surgery center. A slight eighty-nine-year-old gent named Dick specializes in flower deliveries in the Prairie Center. Some of the glass vases are heavy—bigger than his head!—but Dick never wants help. Did he keep in shape during the hiatus by doing pretend deliveries in his apartment, filling a mixing bowl with water and carrying it from room to room? Dick is certainly in prime shape. He grips each vase on two sides and walks in a slow gait across my little lobby to reach the elevator to the inpatient rehab floor. "Hello, Ben!" he says in a hoarse voice as I hit the button for him. He walks as if he is in the main aisle at Westminster Abbey ferrying a gold doodad to the Queen. I get strength just from watching Dick. Everyone at the center does. He goes to the gym daily. He's a hero to all. "Hello, Dick!"

A scrawny blond prisoner from the state penitentiary, where the virus toll has been high, arrives with an armed guard in a bulletproof vest. It's a stunner—the bright orange jumpsuit, leg irons, wrist irons, *and* handcuffs—but I get out "Good morning" as usual, and request that they both lean toward the gizmo, fitting their heads into the green-dotted outline of a skull.

"Success . . . Success . . . ," Ernie drones in his inimitable tone-deaf way. Then trouble. I must place a band around an arm already encircled twice by metal and then band the weightlifter guard's Atlas wrist. The challenge is attaching the sticky end of the slick strip to the unsticky end. Slips happen, many in each case, as nervousness concentrates in my fingers trying to accomplish the manipulation. They stare seriously as I fumble. Almost as surreal is banding a Parkinson's sufferer. To get that done, my wrist has to follow the movements of his as if the quiver is contagious, now mine.

March 31
Godsmack, Prunes, and Noodles

I have chosen what to the end of time is to be my parking place out of the hundreds of predawn options in the South Lot. It is in the row closest to the street I cross to reach the Prairie Center. It is in front of a small tree with a trinity of three trunks. Before I exit the Subaru, I gaze at the lit foyer in the distance to see if early patients await me, locked out of the lobby because those doors only slide open for badges before 5:00 a.m. Once a couple from North Dakota was waiting. They had driven hundreds of miles to avoid paying for a motel. "Long drive!" I said. "That's nothing," the man replied. Then I let them in. I, rescuing those locked out in the cold! It had a deep private meaning, and it happened quite frequently.

"Good morning. . . . Good morning. . . . Good morning. . . . Good morning. . . ." Does my amiable mantra make me as tone-deaf as Ernie Temerity? Well, most of the day jobs I've worked have required more cheer in the morning than I have naturally felt, and that very reality spawns a genuine desire to create a mood counter to the internal drone of worries. Jack the custodian and I have talked about this. After he lost two children under the age of ten and his marriage fell apart, he lived in his car for some months. "Why not smile?" He says. "Frowning only makes things worse." For both of us part of pandemic health means not losing the vitality of being nice to others. "Happy Wednesday. . . . Happy Wednesday. . . . Happy Wednesday. . . ."

A nurse rushes in, flushed, telling me it is the first time she has been late in twenty years. She sounds appalled. She is four minutes late. The red-vest volunteer upstairs today is Jerry. For seventy-nine years he dwelled on a farm outside Beresford, South Dakota. After his parents died he worked the land for thirty years. He moved to Sioux Falls a few years ago. He has logged almost 4,800 hours as a volunteer. When he emerges from the elevator pushing a patient, he tells the family member beside him the same thing each time: "Pull the car up. I'll get the wheel-chair as close as I kin."

The daily intercom prayer advises: "Trust in the Lord with all your heart and lean not on your own understanding" (Proverbs 3:5). Was it picked by a nun because in these COVID days "understanding" might include the epiphany that God has no mercy whatsoever? Elevator opens. A muscular rehab specialist exits with a teenage patient who is learning to walk again. The rehab specialist holds the tassel on the safety belt the teenager wears.

I enter the foyer with a spry patient in a suit and tie departing after a colonoscopy. He asks what my Easter plans are. I shrug. He has a delicious plan: making the traditional Good Friday Russian dish of prunes and noodles. Dad and son from Austin, Texas, swagger in unmasked. Dad wears a bandanna over his head, though. They are here to visit a relative on the rehab floor. To jolly them into compliance I mention Austin is a music city I revere. Bandanna describes a cool Godsmack show at Gilley's in Dallas.

Some nurses that clocked in after I did leave long before I do, tossing a goodbye my way. They leave fresher than any nurses I've ever seen leave any unit. Still bouncy. When each reaches the foyer, a hand rises and the mask is ripped off with gusto.

On average I'm distributing five boxes of fifty masks during my eight-and-a-half-hour shift. But some Midwesterners have survived a pandemic without ever wearing one until now. When I explain the mask regulation, they stare like I am a platypus. They don't know to bend the top wire to fit it over the nose or that the blue side faces out.

April 5
Vaxed and Vexed

I learn from 1010 WINS that 100 million Americans have received at least one vaccination. It is a warm darkness as I cross the lot listening to bird frenzy in ornamental trees. By the end of the day we'll be near ninety degrees. I touch the badge clipped to my shirt. Still there, with its strip that triggers the sliding door to open before 5:00 a.m. I'll get in.

The surgery list I get from the fourth-floor clerk indicates twenty-one procedures today. She is always cheerful ("How are you, Ben?"), though she arrives at 4:00 a.m. Her car is the only car in the immense lot when I get there. I love her name: Rainy. For a half hour we are the only staff below the fifth floor. Back in the lobby I open a desk drawer and remove serrated sheets of the day's color of band (yellow). There are twenty bands to a sheet. I separate singles while listening to Edward Elgar playing on the phone. A skewed heap of bands collects next to my thermos of coffee. Desk height makes me feel like I am a *Wind in the Willows* creature in a nest doing domestic chores—Ratty preparing to meet an honored guest, Mole.

Enter the nurse known as the Maskless Dotless Wonder because he refuses to wear a mask in the lobby, never bows to Ernie. Is he high? He makes farting noises with his lips like a restless five-year-old as he waits for the elevator. Enter the Fly Boy Bakery delivery person carrying the wide white box with the cellophane lid. The colonoscopy walk I am beginning to recognize. It's a jerky gait upon arrival, and upon exit a decided creep, cup of water clutched. I've had the procedure. The ordeal is the preparation. Drinking the liquid that seems to purge you of all your human stains, but at the price of making you feel like you are drowning in them.

At 7:04 a.m. the parking-lot lights blink off. Dawn. I watch telephone wires slink into view, the crosses of the poles.

Today's volunteer is laconic Eunice. She was born in Jasper, Minnesota. Her white tennis shoes are bigger than her feet could be: good for balance. She's at least eighty. Each time she appears in the lobby she asks in an alto voice: "Keeping busy down here?" Like all volunteers she receives an eight-dollar cafeteria voucher for each shift—a treat for a person living on a fixed income. She takes her meal home to make it last.

For the first time, I page a valet to park a car idling outside the foyer. I tear the ticket in half, give the top half to the patient, the bottom to a hulking green-jacketed valet out of a village short story by Frank O'Connor. Brian splices his sentences together with a friendly gurgling sound, red cheeks bumping thick eyeglasses. When paged he rushes with a straight back, but knees bent, so that he looks like a man seated on a stool who is also running.

At 2:42 p.m., after work, from RN Ryan, I receive the first shot of the Pfizer vaccine at a drab one-story building hospital administrators have tried to lend spiritual gravitas by naming Pasque Place after the early spring flower in the buttercup family with the name that means Easter in French. To reach

Ryan I check in at one table in a spacious carpeted room, then bring paperwork to another table. The clerk behind the second desk takes my filled-out form, glances at it, glances up at masked me, asks, "Are you Hispanic?" I know the CDC is collecting demographic data but . . . I checked White on the form. Does she think I have lied for some reason? Did not understand the question? Is she unsettled by my pile of dark hair? Practicing to be a poll watcher asking the same question in 2022? America on edge. "Why do you ask?" I ask. She does not—or cannot—explain. I move on to my serum dose, the fifteen-minute observation period.

Folding chairs are spaced out, facing various directions. It's quiet like we're strip-mall churchgoers in a congregation that lacks a unifying belief in a deity. Tank tops (since it is now above ninety degrees). Shorts. Leggings. Sandals. Most tap smartphones. I read the printed-out obituary of author Beverly Cleary, dead at age 104. Fifteen minutes up, I leave holding the fact sheet for the Pfizer-BioNTech vaccine. The last ingredient listed in the recipe is sucrose or table sugar. Anne gets her second shot tomorrow.

April 6
The Oil Man

Today's volunteer I think of as the Oil Man, due to his tale about recently selling the Nebraska oil company his family started in 1931. Did he move here because the state's tax and banking laws are exceedingly friendly to the rich—so friendly that dictators from foreign countries conceal profits in Dakota trusts, according to the Pandora Papers? The business involved trucking Texas and Pennsylvania crude to Omaha to mix with additives for the ag industry. The Oil Man has tried to incite political conversations by making certain side comments, but I've wiggled into an easier topic each time because I do want to keep liking him. He has the quaint idea I am someone who drinks only herbal tea. He is a ball to watch and listen to as he wheels out dazed patients in no shape for a conversation but having one anyway. "Your son-in-law seems very nice." Nod. "Glad to have it over with, aren't you?" Nod. "Going to go home and take a nap? Have breakfast at the Original Pancake House? Sausage?" Nod. The Oil Man is famed for obsessively sanitizing wheelchair handles, elevator buttons. He forces on Rainy a crude concoction involving vanilla coffee creamers, coffee, half-and-half, packets of Sweet'N Low. He has asked me if I want "a special," and I've gotten out of that too.

When I return from my break, carrying the thermos of coffee and a Styrofoam cup of water, O'Connor the valet in his humming voice jests: "Two-fisted drinker, eh?"

As I've been doing since I started, I ask each arriving patient and their companions: "Have you had any COVID symptoms?" Today I do not get beyond "Have you . . ." before a man replies, "No . . . no . . . to all your questions." I hear his exhaustion with the plague. I feel my own exhaustion with the routine. But, I think, exhaustion will not stop the virus from replicating, and exhaustion is not equivalent to the absorption of events. Recent history has not even begun to be absorbed by cultures yet. Even if there were not a single new infection, these epidemic echoes are going to go on and on and on.

A radiology employee races into the lobby, escaping her department. Trouble: there has been a cyberattack on the ELEKTA software that directs the gamma knife beam to exactly the right spot. A patient with a cancerous eye is on the table in position for treatment that can't be delivered. The waiting room is packed with other patients scheduled for today. "System-wide attack," she says. Then: "Maybe I'll get a day off!"

April 7
"Are You Still Writing Down Sayings?"

On the commute I notice headlights of vehicles on South Cliff Avenue spilling over the stones in Woodlawn Cemetery. Polished granite and marble slabs gleam like computer screens planted in the earth above dead users. Ice-white shimmers.

I set my backpack on the desk chair, turn, and receive a scolding from a pink sticky note on the desktop: PLEASE DON'T PUT OUT AS MANY STAFF DOTS. WE HAD TO WASTE A LOT ON TUESDAY. There's a cost-cutting evaluator of dot usage? Aye-aye. Did I go overboard because each dot potentially represents a hospital worker with no fever? Was it a fantastical effort to create—out of decals—more health in a state where the COVID numbers are climbing and Governor Noem is MIA?

Andrew, a hyperpolite young man in a lemon polo shirt who screens visitors at the Prairie Center main entrance, says all screeners are going to be fired in late May, regardless of the virus infection rate. He is the master of presence. The unseen part of his masked face is somehow reflected in prisms of hazel eyes. Andrew gone? Not nice.

"My husband is coming home!" a lobby visitor in a special outfit exclaims on her way up to the rehab floor. Soon it happens, a procession in the most common order: wife leading a husband in a wheelchair being pushed by a nurse, followed by a second nurse pushing a cart laden with flowers and belongings that range from books to framed photos. Wife goes for the car. Car pulls under the carport, loading happens, and they are gone, pointed toward home, a new start after a near-death experience. A bell is rung in the unit when someone leaves, reminding the rest it is possible.

A strapping executive in a dark suit, blue shirt, and satiny tie charges in and pivots to exit through the door to the atrium, when I fire a "Good morning!" at his heart. He stops. He turns. I met him once at the eICU. It's the CEO of the hospital organization. He is not a doctor. His expertise is human resources. When he was anointed by the sisters, he composed a chummy letter to employees that mentioned his stint as a singing waiter in Vermillion, South Dakota, when he attended college there. "How are you today!?" he yells. It's a warning, a warning that I better be "Wonderful!"

The next whoosh of the door ushers in the final surprise of the shift. A nurse from the eICU materializes in a fury of shampooed bangs, lipstick, vibrant polyester. She was the one who cried "Gotcha!" with verve upon identifying a charting error by another RN. I have not seen anyone from the unit since I worked a last night shift in April of 2020. "One of my favorite ICU nurses," I say. I liked her outward energy. How she spent a half hour sanitizing her telehealth station as the pandemic dawned. I admired her adherence to treatment protocols, no exceptions. She'd challenge a drowsy eICU doctor at 2:00 a.m. She had the seniority. She started in telehealth when telehealth started here: 2004. Most of all, I valued her wacky sense of humor. When I invented the Silver Moon Lotion Bar and the Last Chance Lotion Bar, she—Imagine Dragons fan—pounded pump handles to sample lemon elm goo and mango mud cream and the Jergens and the Bronner's and the limited-edition Dead-Sea mineral gunk. Then she'd rub and rub and rub her hands together, wide grin admiring the confused reek ringing her. Nothing made me, proprietor and lotionista, happier. These whimsies helped keep us human during the numbing virtual health care shifts involving multitudes of electronic-medical-record systems connected to the thirty-six different hospitals the telehealth staff of five supported during each twelve-hour shift.

Gotcha is my age. A cancer survivor, she receives infusions at the Prairie Center to ward off another bout. On summer

Sundays she and her husband park their Caddy in the parking lot of Hardee's like other baby boomers with buffed vintage cars. She yodels my name. Her earrings are opulent like fruit on a French chandelier. "Are you still writing down sayings?" She loved it that I cared enough to take notes during shifts as a way of better understanding the telehealth setting. Does she mistakenly think I am writing a soon-to-be-best-selling novel just about her blazing collars? She began her career in the 1980s in Hawaii at a hospital where a patient leaped from an upper hospital window, landing softly on an awning below. "Still at it," I respond. "Good!" As she exits I recall another of her signature sayings: "Yepper!" for yes. She was disliked for always being right by Nurse Hot Mess, Nurse Buckaroo, tattooed Nurse Nichole, Nurse Carrie, Nurse Sparks, and others who preferred not to be on the receiving end of "Gotcha!" Besides me the only one who could easily tolerate Gotcha was Nurse Judith, a former nun, who sipped the dandelion tea.

April 9
Garnished Wages

Today my first check is finally supposed to be auto deposited, but no money goes in because the entirety of the check is garnished to pay for the company health plan I fell behind paying for when I had no income for two months. On May 1, when our Affordable Care Act plan begins, this robbery will end—the cost cut from over $600 a month to an income-based payment of less than $100. What to do until then? I e-petition HR for a payment from a hospital-foundation fund that assists employees in financial emergencies, some, like this one, caused by hospital policies.

April 12
Ghostbusters

First light sneaking into the lobby reveals soap smears on sliding glass doors. These specters on glass are considered scandalous. First a waddling manager of cleaning examines stains left by a weary substitute night-cleaning crew. Waddle wears the rumpled button-down, no tie. You could hide a career behind the megacoffee he carries. He reports what he sees to a higher up. That Ghostbuster struts in (rumpled with tie and aviator specs), squints, grimaces. "Nobody has taken care of that yet? What's going on here? If you ever see anything similar, you let me know." I promise to.

For the first time I notice visitors using Ernie Temerity's flat face as a mirror to groom themselves. Both are men. For the first time I realize why some patients do not move after Ernie chants "Success . . ."—just stand, befuddled. They are hearing impaired. Today a visitor, after being labeled a "Success," approaches my desk, extends her wrist, announces: "Here to see my husband in inpatient rehab. I got out of quarantine today!" Yikes. I band her while leaning away from her as if surfing, catching an invisible virus wave. "Three out of five in our family got it!" Got it, without getting it that you do not behave like this if you got it. After she steps on the elevator, I pat the double mask I never remove in here. To drink I stick a straw up it.

Late in the day—my day, about 1:00 p.m.—I am summoned to HR to retrieve a check from the hand that giveth after taking away. I pass the waterfall spitting scuzzy foam and litter. I reach Plaza 4 and what is currently my least-favorite waiting room in the urban Midwest. I place hands on knees.

Am I ashamed? I recall how my father, the downtrodden lawyer with few clients, resisted applying for food stamps though our fridge was empty, forcing my mother and me to visit drunk grandfather's house, crossing the rattling grates of the Government Bridge over the Mississippi River on a mission. If we took the old thug's abuse long enough—curses, threats to cut children out of his will, raving praise for "Dutch" Reagan (he'd palled around with Ronald Reagan's dissolute brother Moon in Dixon, Illinois)—the beast could be counted on to burst into tears and pry a twenty from the sagging pocket of his plaid bathrobe flecked with ashes and snot. Trickle-down economics. No, I'm not ashamed of arranging for legitimate help for Anne and me. Yes, I'm getting sick of hospital financial hijinks. Finally the check arrives. I rush into Dakota wind that is both refreshing and upsetting.

April 13
Jerry's Fall

Departing for work at 4:15 a.m. is getting more complicated due to the ways the neighborhood of tightly bunched houses has changed since the pandemic's advent.

At one end of our crowded block DEADBEAT has been spray painted on porch windows. Across from our 1916 home with the fireplace is the house I had seen a kid carrying an orange street pylon into last year. Now that place has plywood boards for windows, a plywood door. Each time I see the arrangement I recall the ragged piece of particle board that for many years plugged the hole in the front door of 15 Crestwood Terrace after the day my brother threw our little sister Mitzi clean through glass. They had been arguing on the porch. She landed inside on a bed of shards. He wanted something she wasn't giving him. I saw it, heard it, could do nothing.

Pylon coveter still lives at the plywood-door address, plus his brother—recently released from prison after serving a sentence for cooking meth—and their mother who screams obscenities at them. (She's rangy like Julia Child.) We've been told that her husband—father of the boys—hanged himself in the garage out back. After midnight vehicles park in front of this address that resembles a two-story coffin for those experiencing a living death. Friends? customers? dart in, dart out. Sometimes people sleep in the cars out front. Sometimes people pound on the plywood, receive no answer, and just stay, sitting on the steps for hours. *Imagine being in such bad straits that your hope lives there!* Sons fight in the yard and the mother calls the police and they come and boys run and police go. Or the three align to drive away a rough friend? customer? One night a girl in the yard cried: "God, please kill Dylan's baby!" Dylan is the former inmate. Daily, before dawn, a silver tanker full of milk thunders down our street, heading toward the silos of the Land O' Lakes facility beside the railroad tracks.

After locking the front door, I move as fast as possible to the garage and when in the car lock it quick before turning the key, backing out. I'm panting.

Before 5:00 a.m. I let into the lobby a masked woman who cooks for the surgeons. "What's on the menu today?" I ask. Cuisine: one of my favorite topics. "Lasagna," she replies. I have not been able to talk lasagna with anyone in a *long* time! "What brand of ricotta do you use?" "Oh, I don't use ricotta. It's too strong. I use cottage cheese."

I notice volunteer Jerry approaching the foyer in an overcoat. Dogged, he walks—very deliberate steps—then falls. I see him go down. As he falls he turns so that he hits the pavement with his shoulder. I rush out. Stroke? Heart attack? He fell slow but heavy. Seeing his descent was like seeing a generation fall—the generation COVID felled—but Jerry, he is not dead when I get to him. He is rustling. Grumbling. "Help me up," the old farmer commands. His lips are the same bloodless hue as the rest of the skin on his face. Eyes like flecks of paper peeling off a highway billboard. "Come on, grab on!"

I extend my hand toward his reaching hand. Our fingers entwine. I lean back, a weight for Jerry to pull against. He squeezes. I feel power, not weakness—a force to want to attach to. It's like I'm getting a massive transfusion of Jerry's rural history— the determination, the wherewithal, the modesty that dictates the ethic of charity be well concealed under a gruff demeanor. As I pull he pulls, and the South Dakotan begins to raise like a barn, neck veins surfacing in a woodgrain pattern.

Once he is upright, I walk close by his side in case he starts to go down again. ICU's are full of men his age who have fallen. Do not want Jerry to go down again. As the lobby door whooshes open, I ask him again if he is alright. He insists he is. After he boards the elevator I debate calling upstairs to warn the staff that he fell—"Look out for Jerry"—but I conjecture he would not like nurses paying special attention. He'd like me to be the only one who knows. He's independent and dignified. A few times he reappears in the lobby, pushing a young patient as his own side throbs from the tumble. "Pull the car up. I'll get the wheelchair as close as I kin." On one occasion he deviates from his trusty tune. After getting a patient to the car, he attempts to explain what happened. It's tough. He's shy. In hesitating sentences that melt into a mumble, he tells of a knee he had replaced, and the inability to lift the repaired leg as high as the other, and. . . . He's telling me what I already know: he's hardly through.

April 14
The Gaits of Dawn

Exactly a year ago I discharged to DEATH in eCare Manager the first COVID fatality connected to the local Smithfield Foods factory: Agustín Rodríguez. I think of that worker often, and his widow Angelita: "I lost him because of that horrible place. Those horrible people and their supervisors, they're sitting in their homes and they're happy with their families. In the name of Jesus Christ, these people need to face justice."

Every passing week, employees I greet—nurses and technicians who have served throughout the course of the scourge—are becoming more distinct despite the pleated curtains of the masks in some cases, and in others because they enter not wearing a mask, allowing a brief glimpse of a complete face before protection is strapped on.

Lanky, goateed male nurse in purple Minnesota Viking shorts and matching hoodie no matter what the weather, hands stuffed in pockets, torso leaning forward. Nurses in Sturgis motorcycle-rally gear or star-spangled leggings. The nurse with the Notorious RBG T-shirt and the jazzy nurse from Kansas City and the nurse who asks, "How is your family, Ben?" and the other one who often asks, "How is your writing going, Ben?" Nurses have to excel in the art of asking to do their jobs well, mastering different tones to fit different situations and different people, and asking not only in words but with hands, necks, and eyes. Even before a shift, they are at it. All of them change into aqua scrubs in the locker rooms upstairs.

In the predawn lobby I feel like a lighthouse keeper looking out for ships of faces. Young sleepy nurses with young children that kept them up yawn "Good . . . morning" and alpha nurses wish me "Good morning!" before I can greet them. They will become managers of nurses in no time. Marathoners who pace themselves and mouth *Hello* rather than speaking. Newbies with those eyes. Judgmental Jesse, the RN who refers to people as either "evil" or "good." Having no days off in more than a year has backed him into a Bunyanesque allegorical mindset. The nurse who tells me it is on his bucket list to visit . . . Iowa City. (Well, it is the Greenwich Village of Iowa.) The brightly attired community outreach specialist and soccer club founder Moses Idris who, as a youth, spent ten years in an Ethiopian refugee camp after his family fled the civil war in Eritrea. Nurses carrying steel drink containers full of ice clicking like dice in a casino cup. The rehab administrator who delivers such good hugs people bring her depressives to squeeze in the parking lot. The patient care technician who calls Thursday "Friday Jr." Volunteer Dick's sidekick Donna, who is somehow half the size of diminutive Dick but has a voice twice as loud. The nurse who arrives with wet hair because she can't find her umbrella in the house she just moved into. The nurse who each night on the commute home to Salem calls her mom, eighty-two, and dad, eighty-six, who still live on the farm. The volunteer who flaps her arms while tweeting about the heroism of Dorothy Day.

The fogged staff member lenses as if we are in a steam bath at a private club for the myopic. The taciturn volunteer who adds "per se" to the end of sentences as in "At least the wind is not blowing per se." The Romanian medical physicist who quips "Bonjour!" at me and gets "Bonjour Monsieur!" back. Today the valet out of a Frank O'Connor story is wearing a Nike cap when he arrives. It doesn't belong in an O'Connor story. And the dreamy custodian who checks in with me a few times each shift asks if I might bring him back a little souvenir from New York City the next time I visit. "Sure, Jack. What would you like?" "Wind chimes." "Wind chimes?" "Wind chimes."

A woman who has had a lumpectomy is pushed into the lobby. She asks questions about showering while her husband gets the car. The nurse's instructions are clear, the patient thanks her, and thanks her. This is the brilliance of good nurses, a big life based on the integrity of an endless succession of small things done right for others.

April 21
"Chop Chop!"

As I roll into the South Lot, the velvety voice of WQXR's Nimet Habachy—a disk jockey I first heard thirty-six years ago—announces she is next going to play the last four songs Richard Strauss composed: "Spring," "September," "When Falling Asleep," and "Sunrise."

It is the day after the guilty verdict in the Minneapolis trial of Derek Chauvin, the police officer who executed George Floyd. Selwyn Jones, Floyd's uncle, lives in Gettysburg, South Dakota, where he owns a motel. When a reporter asked if the news had "brought him any closure," he responded: "No. Because I'm so obsessed with making the change and not seeing any Black man . . . not getting a fair shake because they are Black." Mr. Jones recently led the successful effort to remove the Confederate flag from the shoulder patch on the town's police uniform.

The verdict isn't mentioned during the shift. Nor is there mention of the other news too heavy for casual conversation—a well-respected nurse killed during a bow-hunting accident, shot with an arrow by his son in a field. The pair were after turkeys.

Husband of an arriving patient at first refuses to bow to gizmo, saying, "I got my temperature taken online." "That can't be," I reply. He points, voice rising. "Shut up! This place almost killed me last week. You shut up!" His emaciated partner stares, huddling inside a baggy hoodie. "I'm sorry, I know it's a hassle but. . . ." "I said shut up!" He stomps over to the screen, sways in front of it, bows too deeply, unbows, groans to let me know how much distress he is in, does manage finally to elicit "Success!" then stomps back to the desk I stand behind. I've banded his partner. He draws back his fist. He's got short arms. I don't think he can reach me. The jab is straight and it stops well short, a theatrical way of offering up his limb to the band I pinch. "Chop chop!" he yells. Will he grab and twist my wrist when I try to do my job? He does not. He keeps shouting: "Chop chop!" to rattle me. It works. After these darlings are in an ascending elevator, I go over how I handled the situation. What might have dees-calated the situation? Don't want my heart thrumming like this again in here.

Mr. Chop's eyes were all over the place. I wasn't a person to him. But it's not just that warring pandemic factions are blind to each other. Seeing others cannot happen until you see enough of yourself to have a good idea of who you are.

COVID numbers rising at Washington High School in Sioux Falls. Eight deaths reported in the twenty to twenty-nine age group in South Dakota. Three million global deaths.

April 22
Medicine of Hopper

On the dark drive to work, fruit-tree blooms are like angel food cakes balanced on tables of branches. Across the street from the forsythia-bush border of Woodlawn Cemetery are stairs to a second-story apartment. Security light blasts painted steps. Each commute, when I glance at the austere tableau, I'm reminded of the paintings of Edward Hopper. His colors and strokes reveal sublime depths of personality in the simplest of structures. The windowsill. The bed frame. The palladium curtain.

When I arrive, before doing anything else, I apply a screen-ing dot to the thermos tin cup. Next time someone has a lobby tantrum, I'm going to point at that dot, and say: "You think you have it bad!? Even Stanley the thermos had to have his tempera-ture checked." It will work. It will knock them off message and it will work.

Over weeks I've cultivated another approach to less fraught situations of mask antipathy. When an unmasked person enters and ignores the table where the free masks are available, I don't say anything for a minute. Then, after we've exchanged a few pleasantries, I ask: "Do you have a mask of your own? Or would you like one of ours for free? Take as many as you like."

There's nothing I can do to calm the visitor who recoils at the sight of the elevator. "There are no stairs I can take!?" Her eyes are desperate. Her husband does not look surprised. "There must be stairs." I don't know of any that patients have access to and tell her that. "I can't take an elevator. I can't!" Currently the tallest building in South Dakota is eleven stories. Is it that she has never been in an elevator before? "I'll find someone to take me the back way!" She exits the lobby in search of assistance. "My wife had a bad fall as a child," her empathetic husband, the patient, explains.

Immensely pleasurable young bunny sighting during my break snack at the base of atrium grandeur. Hop, hop, hop on mulch piled around evergreen bushes. I sit between the two indoor waterfalls. One stream of recirculating water descends in front of Rost Meditation Room stained glass. The other cascades beside bronze statues of tykes in galoshes and raincoats, carrying umbrellas.

April 23
The Battery

The phone dings as I am replenishing the table mask supply again. It's a message from Brooklyn-born Ivan: "Happy Friday!" I like the actuality of my Prairie Center lobby and his PNC bank lobby on Seventh Avenue communicating. We keep learning new things that we have in common. For instance, Battery Park, the heel of Manhattan, with its view of the Statue of Liberty and Ellis Island, has played a formative role in both our lives. After his marriage broke up, he retreated there to stand at the rail and gaze at the grace of open water. When I worked at the library of the New York Stock Exchange while attending night classes at NYU, I lunched in the park, buying a seventy-five-cent potato knish, and picking at the damp crust of the heavy treat while observing orange Staten Island ferries, tire-strung tooting tug-boats, and gulls plucking at their sustenance. I never tired of the view. I'm equally enthralled by the shifting dunes of clouds I see from the lobby desk. Lives in transition grow watchful to keep from going wrong.

April 26
Socially Distanced Pickle Spears

Irresistible zest of the frequent visitor to the rehab floor who calls her husband "Babe" and brings him pecan sticky rolls and other things he should not eat. She sports an antic white bale of hair. Grimy flag masks and voluminous gaiters (neck bunting) follow on her cantering high heels. The flags do not match. Some are black, white, and blue. Others black, white, and red. Some are just gray. Or involve a snake.

Patient, ninety-four, upright, not even a cane, and accompanied by a son leaning on a walker. I meet a retired waitress who for many years authored the relish trays at the Knotty Pine Steak House in Elkton, South Dakota. The Sappho of salt. We used to drive out there before the pandemic. Built in 1947. Cabin timbers beside Highway 10. Parking lot surrounded by cornfields. The tantalizing relish tray featured herring, port-wine cheese spread, pickles, black and green olives. She says the place has reopened with spaced tables and other safety measures in place. "They're doing a good job with that." Are the pickle spears socially distanced? I wonder idly. I ask about the jukebox. Still there, dusty hood thrust open, stacked vinyl innards exposed. Sometimes the only way to play discs by Dion and Chuck Berry is to place them manually on the turntable.

Receive second Pfizer shot at Pasque Place. This time my ethnicity is not questioned.

April 27
Mask Amnesia

Morning intercom prayer begins: "Please, God, help restore the MOSAIQ program." Did I hear that right? I heard it. When IT has to resort to prayers it's a problem.

A nurse wheels an unmasked patient out of the elevator, catching her error halfway across the lobby. "Oh, I forgot to have you mask up before you left the room! Here. . . ." She runs to the table, gets the patient a mask. "What's wrong with me?" the nurse laments. A pandemic phenomenon I christen "mask amnesia." Seeing someone masked so much during a day that you see them masked even when they are not.

April 28
The Adventures of Sir Signmeister

Vice president of hospitality bursts into the lobby when less than ten minutes remain in my shift. He's the big suit who has been threatening to cut the valets—Nike O'Connor among them, Nike O'Connor told me. His gaze demands I listen. I obey. "Do we need this SCREENING QUESTIONS sign? No! What about this one?" Questions in Spanish. "It's the same sign as the sign over there." Uh-huh. Redundancy is the foe he combats redundantly. He is talking very fast using the same phrases in many orders. Is he stable? He rips down FACE MASK REQUIRED BEYOND THIS POINT signs that have congregated in the foyer and around the door to the atrium. "Six signs are less effective than one!" he declares, nodding, drunk on sign eradication, spinning closer to my desk before pivoting to point at the MAKE SURE DOOR CLOSES FULLY sign on the Radiology Department staff entrance. "You put this here?" he accuses. "No." "Well, we don't need it. And don't put it back up after I'm gone. Don't get sneaky. We've got to clean this place up. Look at that trash basket of yours." Packed with a day's discarded masks and the MediChoice boxes they are shipped in. "Empty it!" I nod. "Well, you're new. You're still learning." I nod. I believe people are always telling some truth about themselves, if you can find the crack in all the rest and peer through. I fail in his case. The persecutor of valets and laminated plastic flips me a business card, leaves me with a tale of his valor. Once upon a time during a plague there was a patient who arrived at the hospital and refused to don a mask. He was there to have an MRI. When a concierge failed to convince him to mask up, Sir Signmeister was called. (With a bugle, I imagine.) Mask resister explained that at the start of the epidemic he had gotten down on his knees, asking for God's protection. Sir reminded the resister he was free to go to the other hospital in the city for the test, but that there, too, he would be asked to mask. Sir wondered aloud if the MRI was really necessary, and when assured it was important, very important, Sir quoted Apostle Paul to the resister. He reenacted, a stage whisper: "In humility count others more significant than yourselves." Signmeister's brow smiled a smile that made me want to offer him a toothpick. Patient had his MRI, hospital got its $3,000. I leave twenty minutes late.

May 5
Nurse D and Eternity

Recently released statistics indicate the birthrate in America fell by 4 percent in 2020, the biggest drop in fifty years. The CDC issues a report linking last summer's Sturgis motorcycle rally in South Dakota to 649 COVID cases in twenty-nine states.

If an outsider knew only one thing about this state, it was likely the Sturgis rally held in a western area of the state called the Black Hills. But bearded nihilists astride lowriders, often pictured (or imagined) in the news, did not represent the real-life complexities at play in this pandemic drama. There were biker nurses, biker teachers, biker dentists, bikers employed by Volunteers of America and the Good Samaritan Society. Sturgis was old-home week for Dakotans. Participation went back generations. The superspreader calculus was harder to take seriously if your comfort level with an environment went that deep—and breaking the chain of attendance was scarier than a threat you could not see. In addition to the virus, Sturgis bred music concerts, picnics, Spearfish Canyon scenic group rides, and—like any human gathering—language. "Sturgis surprise" meant an unplanned pregnancy connected to campground celebrations. I learned it when I worked at the aquatic center. A rattled teenage lifeguard reported for work right after finding out about her "Sturgis surprise" and went around telling everyone she ran into on the pool deck, including me, adding she had "yet to tell her mother."

In honor of National Nurses Day, staff in the surgical unit receive aloe vera plants, a botanical with proven medicinal qualities. I help carry boxes of pots to the unit as I think of estimable eICU nurses surrounded by tall screens linking them to the pulses of patients in trouble at tiny hospitals in places like Spirit Lake, Iowa, and Gillette, Wyoming.

Nurse F, who booked a fiftieth wedding anniversary cruise for herself and her husband, only to cancel it when he went on another gambling binge. She requested a divorce at last. She invited her beloved ten-year-old granddaughter to sail to Finland.

I met soft-spoken Nurse D's son when he visited the eICU to have lunch with his mother. He was then about to earn an MA in physics from an Ivy League school. After that happened he enrolled in a PhD program in Colorado. Toward the end of the first semester he hit a tree while skiing, spending days on a ventilator before being unhooked because he was brain dead. Would Nurse D come back? everyone wondered. After a period of mourning, she did, spending shifts tending to vented patients the same age as her son. Fentanyl ODs. I-90 crash victims. How could she bear it?

She bore it. This was her chosen career. She functioned exactly as before—one of the best nurses in the unit—except that now when she asked me to discharge a patient that had perished on her watch, she would text me: "He is celebrating his birthday in eternity," a phrase derived from a quote by the Roman philosopher Seneca that goes, "The day which we fear as our last is but the birthday of eternity." I still had a lot to learn from Nurse D. I missed working with her. When she discovered we had a Montmorency cherry tree in our yard she asked for seeds and I brought her some.

A rumor is circulating that the eICU will soon be sold to a for-profit holding company.

May 6
Lego Guy

I see him again during my break. This means I wasn't hallucinating the first time I spotted the spindly, middle-aged cancer patient in a New England Patriots jacket that on his frame looks like a robe. He is bringing Lego creations with him to show the Prairie Center staff. He is balding. Wire-rim glasses, khakis. He rushes across the sidewalk—literally running to receive chemo like maybe nobody on earth does except him. Any sickness the therapy causes is hardly rivaled by the joy he takes in bonding with nurses and volunteers. Do the mass of men now lead lives of quiet loneliness rather than quiet desperation? Male desperation has gotten louder—it's all over social media—but loneliness is always a soft-shoe dance. He transports creations on a tray. From a distance this one looks like a wedding cake. It is not a cake. A battleship with tiers? A castle? Does he use appointments here as a deadline to finish projects? The first time I saw Lego Guy, in a waiting room, the tray was balanced on a forearm as he spouted details about his latest plastic tank to a circle of volunteers and nurses straining to relate. "That's interesting." "You don't say. . . ." "I like the blue with the red."

In the last twenty-four hours there have been 414,000 new COVID cases in India—the current global hot spot. An internal email informs staff that over 9,000 South Dakotans are past due for a second dose of the Moderna or the Pfizer vaccines. A patient from Pipestone, Minnesota—home of oldies station KISD and the sour cream–raisin pie at Lang's—reaches the lobby and slumps into a brown chair, waiting for his wife who is parking the car. "At first when I heard about people refusing the vaccine I was upset, crying . . . now I think *let them die.*" He stops talking. He is crying again.

May 10
Powers That Might Be

For the first time since February of 2020 the New York Public Library allows in-person browsing at ninety-two branches. We've made a leap of faith and booked two seats on a June flight to New York City to see Anne's parents and a few dear friends.

Into the foyer Eunice pushes a wheelchair filled by a man twice as wide as she is. When she returns, I comment: "You could probably lasso a tornado if you wanted." She replies: "Oh, I wouldn't get that carried away." We laugh. This program of volunteers is brilliant. The volunteers are half a friend, half a coworker. Apart in a good way from the grid. It relaxes everyone. It takes the aging out of aging.

A member of the Lakota Nation advocates for COVID inoculations as she sits in the lobby waiting for a ride. She talks of the toll taken on her nation by diseases of "white men invaders" and the tragedy that her people "had no protection" against illnesses like smallpox imported from Europe on ships. . . .

May 11
"Orange Blossom with Hints of Sage and Lemon"

A nurse who for months had no sense of smell due to COVID regales me with a description of walking through a cloud of a colleague's perfume in the South Lot.

May 17
Farm Reports and Subway Schedules

Station 1010 WINS reports around-the-clock F-train service has resumed in New York City, and the end of the midnight Manhattan restaurant curfew. Whenever a street or park or building is cited in a news story, I try to picture it as I last saw it. *The West Fourth Street F platform below the A platform, both poised at the end of a tiled pedestrian tunnel where musicians strum the Rasta songbook or wail Dylan poetry—a tunnel gently descending from the station entrance next to the basketball court. Those turnstiles I used to bump with my hips like I was dancing with them.*

I am informed corn is "two leaf high" at some area farms and that "it's wet where we are in Britton but dry all around us." It's a bear to be subjected to excess diligence of any employee anywhere! But without planning to do so, I begin flashing patients the thumbs up after I put them in the elevator, make final eye contact. For fun I tape a handwritten reminder note to the back of my smartphone: *Stop at Hy-Vee after work for a carton of half-and-half.* Technology reversed. Now Ernie Temerity is rumored to be retiring soon. Where will he go? Prague? Fort Myers? The hospital starts allowing two visitors per patient and announces a renewed effort to combat "drug diversion," an epidemic of staff members stealing opioids prescribed for patients.

May 20
"No, I'm Not Ready!"

"Hello folks," I greet two women as they enter the lobby. I ask for the patient's name. Agnes wears the vintage red-and-white dress and good shoes. Her daughter is well-dressed in a more modern style. Agnes's COVID test has come back negative or she wouldn't be here. She has known about the surgery date for weeks or months. Yet she seems stunned to be in the lobby, and settles gingerly into a brown chair, purse on lap, anxious eyes avoiding looking at anyone or anything. Her hair has been done. She wears a watch. The daughter looks at me as I convey that the fourth floor, where the elevator will stop, is not a public area but "the unit itself. You can't get lost." Agnes is eighty miles inside herself. Her stillness is the stillness that requires as much effort as motion. I continue in a soft voice: "Now that you've checked in, you can go on up. Are you ready?" The daughter has taken her mother's hand. I get no response. In an even softer voice I repeat: "Are you ready to go up?" Her head jerks. She's been ignoring me because she's heard me. "No! I'm not ready!" Age has freckled her face. Her eyes glisten like creek stones. I glance at the daughter, who is looking to me for an answer. Every week there are new situations when dealing with the public. What to do? Not knowing, I let a few seconds tick off the clock, before chancing a guess. "Would you like me to go up with you?" Her face relaxes a bit, not enough. "Would you like to take my arm?" She nods, biting her lip. I extend an arm. She rises slowly, purse swinging. Her hand lands on my forearm like a sparrow. We promenade to the elevator. I punch the up arrow. When the silver button is punched, a ring of blue light appears around it. Usually, to lighten the mood, I say, "See the blue ring? It's a mystical thing." But her mood can't be lifted, only borne. That takes ligaments of the concentration she is exerting. I do not want to interrupt again. We step in. I punch the floor number. Another blue ring. Door closes. Daughter is beside us. By now I can feel the chill of Agnes's touch through the thin shirt I am wearing. Her fingers are very cold. There's my childhood history of unwanted touching by strange adults, but this is not perverse, and it is not violent. She is clinging to my arm as if I were made of bone china too.

May 21
The Return of Sir Signmeister

He lopes in wearing the same suit, same smiling brow. He acts in the same compulsive and worrisome fashion that brings three numbers to mind: 911. "What's this? Too much!" He rips down two MASK UP signs. "I took these down last week! What happened?" I don't say a thing. Someone reposted the signs, not me. "Superfluous? We're getting rid of checks soon!" Goodbye SCREENING QUESTIONS displayed on the door to the Prairie Center. The next SCREENING sign he targets, that he must remove, is posted on glass that becomes inaccessible when the sliding door to the foyer swooshes open as he approaches to do his duty. He retreats three steps, door closes, exposing sign, but as he pounces again the door swooshes open again, making sign unavailable. He spits grains of sound. He backs up three steps, door closes. He tries pouncing faster, but the sliding door wins for a third time, like a devoted mother protecting her laminated child from a wolf. "I'll get it, don't you worry," he warns the door. He jumps back. Door closes, exposing delicious young sign. He jumps to the right. He jumps to the left. A ploy to confuse the electric eye? He hesitates. He dives with arm outreached but no go, too slow, strike four. Only because he is upper management he gets more strikes. It is Buster Keaton hilarious, but sobering to think he's in charge of anything. As the swoosh—lunge—fail pattern continues, I think of Kafka again, of Beckett, of bell hooks—experts at depicting what happens when relationships and institutions devolve under pressure but do not dissolve. Tolerance for nonsense rises until nonsense becomes the chief policy—if not the only policy. How can administrators addled by crisis be asked to address it? Survival for them means denial—behaving as if surrounding dysfunction does not matter—but it all matters. Signmeister does get his prey in the end. Sixth try. Tricks door with a stuttering two-step ploy. Slick devil. I must try to give him more credit.

Though the state has now surpassed 2,000 deaths from the virus, it is the masks citizens are set on fighting. "We have clients as mad as a wet hen about the mask thing at the fitness center," a visitor says today. An aged Roger challenges me. "I won't wear one unless *you* put it on me." Large hairy ears. Don't want to. Need to. I fit loops over the rubbery lobes as he rants: "When is this going to end? When!?" He wears the garb of his alma mater—the University of Minnesota.

For the second week in a row the deliverer of soft drinks to the Prairie Center wants to make my day nicer as he exits pushing a trolley loaded with last week's unsold products. "Want an outdated Pepsi or Dew? The expiration date was only the nineteenth."

May 24
"Passed Nothing?"

It's official: after this week no more Ernie and no more dot-management duties. All I'll have to do COVID-wise is replenish the table mask supply. Will that be enough to keep the facility safe? Staff has been advised to self-screen at home and not report to work if running a fever. A worrisome prospect, given the responsibility nurses feel about making shifts. They'll come in sick, coughing, and make a supervisor order them home. Listening to Ernie's swan song—"Success . . . Success . . ."—I wonder what his hobbies are. Does he fish in castle moats for carp? Golf? Crossword puzzles? Will he end up in a Prague café populated with screens on stalks? He might be moving on, but other technology is sure to take his place. We don't have to open doors now or do our own shopping. We don't have to turn a single dial or lift a cast-iron pan. But our hands are learning tools. An education is lost.

In the meantime, more than 300,000 in India have now died of the virus. A volunteer has arrived with gifts for patients. Rocks painted with the words: JOY, LOVE, HOPE.

Patient in farmwear stumbles into the lobby clutching his stomach. Behind him, the exact same height, is his imperturbable wife. She holds his belt to keep him from toppling forward. He makes it to one of the chairs and collapses into it, doubled over. I ask for a name. "Willie," she replies for him. I check the list. Willie is at the right surgical center. "Oh," he whispers, "It hurts so bad." "We're from Wessington Springs," she says, adding, "A two-hour drive." He keeps hurting. She keeps calm. "Willie did the prep for the colonoscopy as instructed, but he didn't pass anything." Drank gallons of that foul fruit-flavored laxative solution and passed nothing!? Not a drop? In other words, he's about to burst. "Stay where you are, Willie, I'll get a nurse to come down right away. She'll help you." Wife now has her hand behind him, fingers hooked around belt to keep him from hitting the floor. "Just hurts," he murmurs in extraordinary fashion. He is not screaming. The tone is confiding, not hysterical. Despite his agony he is managing to be understated: a Herculean act of stoicism. I message the resource nurse. Within minutes, elevator opens, out comes a willowy, blond, middle-aged RN pushing a blue wheelchair. The wife explains to her what she explained to me. "Passed nothing? We'll have to see what the doctor says about that." Nurse slides bloated, whispering Willie into the chair and wheels him into the elevator as wife repeats her mantra: "We're from Wessington Springs."

May 25
The Cowboy

An authentic cowboy steps off the elevator. I've seen none in six years in Sioux Falls. A lot of Rotarians, homeless men, fast-food workers, contractors, mechanics, stay-at-home dads, professors, snowplow operators, IT specialists, crypto hustlers, taxi drivers, gamblers, and a few of those special pale faces representing a flawed power structure that has not expanded like the city's population, but cowboys? No.

He has delivered his brother into the good hands of the surgical center and is on his way to the Quarry Cafe for coffee.

He wears the complete warm-weather wrangling outfit—straw broad-brimmed hat, plaid-pattern western shirt with pearly buttons, jeans, square-toe boots. The sun-chewed skin. Pocket Pall Malls. Returning with a coffee cup in his fist, he lingers, and we talk. He is a team roper on the rodeo circuit. "Oh yeah. I've had my throat crushed by a hoof." And the throat, from looking at it and hearing it, bounced back pretty good. "And I had a brain aneurysm after being stomped and was on life support for four months. But finally I got back to riding, farming, smoking. Then that COVID really kicked my ass last November. I was in the ICU at Queen of Peace for weeks. Docs wanted to vent me, but I said, if that's what you're going to do, I'm leaving. I won't be hooked up to that machine again. And they backed off." Queen of Peace, located in Mitchell, South Dakota, was one of the hospitals served by the eICU. I often spoke to nurses there when they called to solicit a doctor's help with vent settings. It was common for patients to resist invasive ventilation if they had the energy. Pulling out tubes. Threatening nurses. Sometimes they'd be sedated to the point of cooperation. Sometimes they'd have arms and legs restrained. Sometimes they'd leave AMA: against medical advice. If that happens, insurance won't pay a penny of the stay's cost. The cowboy's getting his way via decree made him rarer. He is the first ICU survivor I've ever spoken to—that I know of. "Take care, bud," he tells me. I tell him it's easier when you don't have a habit of jumping off horses twirling a lasso.

May 26
Eclipse of the Flower Moon

At 4:31 a.m. I stand outside the Prairie Center looking at the silvery-blue orb. Wisps of clouds pass beneath like smoke from a campfire angels are sitting around. At 5:07 a.m. I venture out again and see the eclipse is underway, a bite out of a curve of the moon. At 5:27 a.m. that bite is larger, nearly half of the moon in shadow. It brings to mind an X-ray of a sick lung, along with English lace on a mahogany table, a stingy brim hat woven by Bunn of Harlem, a baseball in flight at Yankee Stadium, facets of a Tiffany jewel.

I haven't seen Jolene since our brief training session, but again I think of Jolene. Her daughter, she told me that day, has Alzheimer's disease. Early fifties. Married. Kids.

XXXL warm-up suit, cane, a testicle larger than a basketball . . . but the arriving patient remains in a jovial mood somehow. "Do you need a wheelchair?" I ask. "Get me a fat boy's chair." He chuckles. I get the biggest foyer wheelchair. He shimmies into it. "Here to take care of this big boy," he says, tapping the crotch bulge with a cane. I go bland. It's good to go bland at times like these. "They'll do their best. A crisp unit."

A visitor to the rehab unit enters the lobby cradling a large cribbage board with horns sticking out of it. "What kind?" I ask. "Elk."

June 1
A Reprieve for Ernie!

For the first time I experience what it is like to work in a dotless lobby, and without the mission of asking visitors if they have virus symptoms. New, large foyer signs on tripods are supposed to do that job for me, but I notice few people who enter stop to read them.

A truck crew drove around the hospital campus removing the temp-scanning screens, but they missed this lobby. Ernie Temerity stands now with his flat face against the wall like a punished student. When someone refers to him, I say: "Ernie missed his flight to Fort Myers. Makes you wonder." It did me, at least.

June 10–15
Return to New York

The flight lands at LaGuardia. Anne and I are back. 1010 WINS reports 69.7 percent of New York City adults have received at least one vaccine shot.

We enjoy our first meal out since February 2020 at Frankies 457 on Court Street in Brooklyn, near where we were living when we were married in 1989. We choose a table under a tent out back, ordering a lunch of antipasti, lentil soup, two chilled glasses of Nero d'Avola, a rich Sicilian red wine we favor. It is the waiter's first maskless shift in over a year, and he feels odd enough to mention this. Others at spaced tables sit around us. Every spoonful of soup and sip of wine feels dramatic. It's as if the pandemic has turned dining out into a sacrament for deprived senses.

A Brooklyn friend invites us to join the group that since April of 2020 has been drumming weekly in front of the Cobble Hill Health Center as a way of cheering on COVID patients and stressed staff. Nara, a filmmaker, helped form the Kitchen Sink Band after news reports indicated the center had suffered more pandemic deaths than any other nursing home in the city. She is a lifelong resident of the neighborhood where the center stands. Anne's parents, whom we are staying with, live not far away, in a brick building on Schermerhorn Street with a green awning reading The Montana.

We meet Nara at her address on a short street once inhabited by her Japanese grandparents (Kimi and Bunji) when the neighborhood of Cobble Hill was affordable. Her grandfather was a draftsman and an artist specializing in street scenes. Her grandmother, a pioneering poet, advocated for the rights of Japanese Americans. Her late mother Ikuyo was a progressive architect and her late father Don a painter and inventor of acoustic gear. Nara's documentary *Flat Daddy* depicts the phenomenon of cardboard cutouts that help American children deal with pro-longed absences of parents serving in the military overseas.

She issues Anne and me claves—percussion sticks—to make the good noise with. She says about ten people are still participat-ing: age range four to seventy-five. Usually Nara's husband Tolan, the biomed specialist at New York Presbyterian, participates, but he just had sinus surgery, is not feeling up to it. Before we leave for the gig, he mentions his hospital will be the nation's first to mandate vaccines for employees. He is happy about that. He often walks over the Brooklyn Bridge to the Manhattan hospital. Nara walked with him during the pandemic's darkest days, the Central Park ICU days.

The Kitchen Sink Band gathers a little before 7:00 p.m. at Verandah Place and Henry Street, at the end of a quaint alley across from the brick nursing home's main entrance. I'm sur-prised to see the drums are improvised. Some players will bang on green overturned recycling bins. Others are prepared to thump bike helmets or poles or bottoms of white plastic buckets. One guy clenches a tambourine. At the top of the hour, noise-making commences, accompanied by yelps and clapping.

The sound attracts attention for blocks. A fascinated woman stops, lifts a phone, films. Anne makes her rhythm by thrashing a NO PARKING sign pole. Those recycling bins make the deep-est sound. Trash can lids make the sharpest sound. The buckets rumble. I hold sticks overhead, tapping a repetitive rhythm as my eyes climb the building's facade and its nondescript rows of windows behind which so many remarkable events happened. Minutes into the tumult, a nurse in dark-blue scrubs exits the center, flashes a thumb's up I translate as: *This is still needed. This still helps. Thanks.* She blows us kisses. She crosses arms over her chest: love in sign language. The band's beat is intense like a mob of commingling heartbeats.

Do I see shadows in some of the windows? I think of Cirino, the first acquaintance we lost to COVID. Of Dr. Butler and the veterinary practice she ran on 145th Street until succumbing to the virus, an office renowned in the community for providing care to animals even if the pet owner could not pay. I think of Tom, the Galileo scholar, who died alone in a Bronx nursing home, and of a fifty-seven-year-old hospital employee back in South Dakota, the one who confessed she had never seen anything fascinating in her life but might soon because she and her husband had scheduled a trip this coming October to see the ocean at Hilton Head. Would she make it? As I keep my rhythm—tah, tah-tah, tah, tah-tah-tah, tah—my eyes meet the blue-gray sky.

June 30

The first case of the Delta variant is reported in South Dakota.

LOG 4

Coda Blue

the sun saying hello
and i know the crows will be back.
sometimes, i think maybe,
maybe it won't be today
—Rahele Megosha,
"codependency"

December 29
Three Dead

In the surgery waiting area at the main hospital, where hall-ways intersect, stands the station of its host. Three free-standing Plexiglas panels atop the desk form a booth that jiggles if nudged. I'm in it at the cusp of the Omicron surge. Last month I had scheduled shifts here, where help is needed due to staff short-ages. Time felt right to add hours to the sixteen I worked at the Prairie Center. I had navigated the Delta surge without a cough like Dick, the eighty-nine-year-old volunteer who, I recently noted, wears a hoop earring. Our courtly pirate.

A list of the day's scheduled procedures is sitting in the Kafka booth when I arrive.

It has been provided by registrars seated down the hall at a half-shell counter. These two despise each other. Snipe, snipe, snipe. Each surgical patient checks in with them. Relatives are then directed to supply host with a name and phone number before inhabiting the waiting area crowned by wall-mounted TV screens. It is host's first job to jot a micro descriptor of the family member (e.g., *Twins ball cap*), so they are easier to locate when the surgeon desires to consult after a procedure. Host's last task is the best one: leading relatives to bedside reunions in the post-op area beyond the dueling banjos.

I glance at the procedures list. At the top: "Amputation of the left foot."

There is only one phone-tapping person in the waiting room so far. Inhaling through two masks (cloth over surgical), I slowly peel off winter layers, draping wool jacket over the booth chair, and slinging my lucky blue sweater over that. I extract Stanley, the dot-wearing thermos, from my backpack, plus three bottles of water. I sit in the cheap black chair that does not swivel. I unlock desk drawers with a key slipped off a hook under the desktop. A somnolent start, yes, but nonetheless I'm dreading more than the nearness of Omicron.

It's been like this each time, which is why I won't be back after completing two last shifts. A gentler financial fix needs to be found in 2022.

Part of it is the oppressive effect of spending hours in the booth amid an atmosphere of compounding tension as the waiting area fills with jittery Midwesterners.

Part of it is the annoyance of being called "the police" when I request that a visitor wear a mask over their nose for the safety of others.

And part of it is the nearness of the ICU, located just down the hall, and the way trouble there spills over into each five-hour host tour of duty. A nurse had informed me it was "a little different" deep in the hive of the hospital—different from the human-interest carnival of a lobby on the medical campus's edge—and true it proved to be.

I miss seeing my parked car from the lobby desk. In the Kafka booth the notion of escape is vague. It feels no less imprisoning because it is loose. The best I can do is stand and stretch, impatient to swim after work.

I unlock the three consult rooms across the hall. I peek in each. They are clean.

I retrieve the cell phone that will snag the calls I'm not at the desk to answer. From another drawer I remove slips used to reserve consult rooms and cards that read: WELCOME! We believe each person who comes to us for care is made in God's image. We will care for you with excellence, compassion, and respect. Your patient is in room: _____.

The TV attached high on the pillar in front of the booth is off. I hide the remote in a drawer to make sure the screen remains devoid of screaming *The Price Is Right* and *Let's Make a Deal* contestants that added a grotesque tone to the previous shift.

The hall that leads past the consult rooms is the wider one. Traffic flows and ebbs. Phone-bent ICU night-shift RNs trudging homeward in hunter-green scrubs. Chattering perky nurses arriving. This morning I encounter no ICU faces I know, but last shift I ran into big, strong Samantha, face shield over N95 mask. Once she split her time between this hub and the telehealth ICU.

"Ben! What are you doing here?"

"Three years as a support specialist at the eICU was enough."

"Yes, it was crazy there, wasn't it?"

I got her. She fled too. For her the real ICU, despite its challenges–coffee grounds hung in rooms to absorb smells dying produced, for example—is preferable. She wants to care for palpable patients, not beige shadows on screens and their telltale columns of lab numbers. Samantha brought me a can of chicory back from New Orleans in 2018, a thank you for what I did not exactly know, but I guessed it had to do with little things I'd done to alleviate tension when we were stuck working twelve-hour night shifts with one of the undisciplined nurses telehealth could enable because bedside providers had ultimate responsibility for patient care. Giggling Facebook surfers. Nothing pisses off a good nurse more than a mediocre colleague. Well-timed wisecracks kept 4:00 a.m. fisticuffs from breaking out.

A few months ago the eICU telehealth service was indeed sold to a private equity firm based in London and New York. Sum not disclosed.

Down the wide hall buzzes a short R2-D2-shaped robot charged with delivering narcotics to various spots in the hospital. Since it is the holiday season, the robot has been slathered with snowflake decals. This drug-pushing automaton was implemented after too many staff members succumbed to the temptation to steal opioids. The robot possesses sensors enabling it to adjust for oncoming traffic: stop, veer left, veer right. Perhaps it even knows the Lindy Hop. Visitors who have not seen the robot before are awed. If you've seen it a few times, you hardly notice. How fast technoweirdness comes to seem normal!

Where is Amber of food service? A nice thing about the hive is that it reconnected me to this friendly person who used to work at Hy-Vee supermarket, where Anne and I got to know her. Dark eyeliner around an intent gaze. High-pitched lilting voice. She always brought a full spirit to a stocking job in the aisles. That was a feat to admire, we knew, having worked repetitive jobs that can negate spirit. Seeing Amber during the first shift in early December seemed a good omen, but I hadn't seen her since.

Gowned and harnessed patients out for a wobbly walk pass by. Clinicians pinching reports. Pat and Mark, maintenance men in navy blue. Cleaning ladies in head scarves, and a short woman in sky-blue scrubs, crinkly plastic cap covering her curls. She's a medical waste transporter. Reports to work early at the Prairie Center, then floats.

"Hi, Pam! Nice to see you!"

She smiles under her mask, mouth motion tugging at the tops of her cheeks, making them dance like little puppets. She has the build of a point guard who has played a hundred thousand games in humid Midwest armories. She doesn't waste one movement.

"How are you, Ben?"

I hear the day's first cigarette in her voice.

"Hanging in."

"Do you like it here?"

"You know the old saying . . . home is where the heart is. I miss the Prairie Center."

She groans in recognition, wishes me luck, and motors toward the next mess.

Monotone intercom recites the Pledge of Allegiance. Kitty-corner from the Kafka booth, two seasoned nurses take time to encourage a younger nurse who is upset about how a recent pregnancy has changed her physique. She tells them she tried wearing "the band" for a few months to regain her former form but got sick of it. "Well," says one of the older RNs, "It is our right to look the way we do. Don't be so hard on yourself."

A smocked housekeeper passes between nurses and booth, delivering her lines to all within hearing distance, and no one. "I'm looking for my blue cart. Anyone seen it? I had to borrow one once. I've checked everywhere. If you see my cart that some-one ran off with. . . ."

Patients with family members start arriving, checking in, fill-ing the waiting room.

Surgeries done here are the most complex and perilous. Patients, exiting the elevator, blink as if warding off a gruesome blade of fluorescence suddenly slicing through the bog of antici-pation. I tell all family members the same thing, my latest tune to chirp.

"After the surgery the doctor will quickly consult with you in one of the rooms across the hall. After that consultation there will be a recovery period for the patient that usually lasts about two hours. Then you will be reunited. The restroom is around the corner. There are vending machines down the hall. There is a cafeteria on the ground floor, but if you do leave for more than a few minutes let me know."

I never tire of saying the spiel because it is a new test each time. A test to make the same words heard by different people—to forge in a few seconds a bond of cooperation via tone, rhythm, content. Do not mutter. Speak slow, sure. If I often fail to get the complete message across to preoccupied listeners, well . . . I know failure is quite natural because the task is not easy. This element of the job routine connects tightly to a writing life.

Surprisingly few heavy coats for a zero-degree day. Our old garage door went up and down eleven times before sticking shut and allowing me to depart.

I begin work on a seating chart I'll pass on to the next host at noon. Draw a rectangle to represent the room: *gray hoodie / red bag / hearts on shirt / wool cap greenish / friday on shirt / grayer hoodie / black toothy gaiter / SDSU hoodie blue / MEM on hoodie / big white coffee cup / grayest hoodie. . . .*

I stick a straw up masks, suck water, count streaks of white light, as if they are sheep, on Plexiglas booth panels. Before this assignment, the winner of My Most Desolate Day Job Seating Arrangement Award was the IBM plant in Vermont, where we Manpower temps were forbidden from sitting with "regular" employees in the segregated lunchroom.

SDSU hoodie begins pacing in a tight circle in front of the Kafka booth. Other pacers take longer loops, encompassing the vending machine area.

Waiting people get bored. Waiting people converse haltingly. One thing that the Prairie Center lobby and here have in common is avoidance of talk about the pandemic's progress. There's talk of vaccines—have or haven't, will or won't—but the incredible death toll, no—survivors with long COVID, no—the lessons to be drawn from how institutions responded, no.

The eerie echoless chamber does, though, acknowledge one real tragedy: that COVID headlines swept out of view countless small and large stories deserving of attention. And the non-COVID talk connects to the reality that shoring up society in the pandemic's aftermath will demand citizens become urgently interested in many things other than the virus. But what? The what will make all the difference—mean progress or more disaster.

A man tells the waiting room universe about the time his absent-minded South Dakota mother missed a corner when knitting and produced an oblong afghan eight feet long. Nervous laughter. In another carpeted corner, the talk is agriculture and racial diversity.

"Without the Hispanic community the dairy industry in our area would be in trouble. Usually they don't work in the machine shop. They have no desire to. It's possible the next generation will have the desire. My grandfather started out as an immigrant, too, in the dairy industry. From Holland. Hispanics are hardworking, and family oriented."

It's the month that ambitious Governor Noem continues using $5 million in federal COVID relief funds to promote the fact that the state welcomes tourists who are not vaccinated. It's the month when there are more than seven million views of a Twitter video depicting a promotion at the halftime of a Sioux Falls Stampede hockey game. In it local teachers are seen scrambling on hands and knees to gather five thousand one-dollar bills off the ice to pay for classroom needs they had no other way to fund. The crowd can be heard cheering wildly.

Phone rings. I jump. Heads in the waiting room turn, wanting news. I never know when a call is coming. Callers are nurses in a huff just like when I was the traffic controller and morale lifter at the eICU. When I pick up the receiver, I again nearly identify myself as "Support Specialist Ben," before I swallow, reset, emit "Surgery waiting, host speaking."

First consult request. I place a family member in Room A. Each room contains chairs, a few small tables, lamps, the box of tissues. Into a plastic slot in the door I place the slip on which I've scrawled the name of the surgeon and the patient's first name.

Shortly after I return to the booth a woman in a fuzzy turtleneck has a question.

"Is there a room I can pump in?"

A mother's room. I consult the dueling banjos. Backs to each other, they play their unhelpful tunes, shrugging. "Can't help you with that." "New one on me."

Walking back to the mother waiting beside the booth, clutching her bag, I improvise a plan of action. I lead her to Consult Room C and turn on the light and slip an index card reading IN USE into the door slot. She thanks me. Whew.

I cast a furtive Kafka clerk glance at the waiting room to avoid attracting anxious eyes. Three more family groups have shifted position! I draw arrows on my chart, but too many arrows spoil the soup. There are already many. And too many patients named Kevin and too many patients named Diane and too many relatives wearing gray hoodies. Two family groups are gone. Where? It makes not a whit of sense, but it can feel as hard to keep track of fifteen adults in this confined area as it was monitoring forty racing kids in a large gym when I worked at decrepit Bowden Youth Center in downtown Sioux Falls.

Phone rings. Another consult room request. I lead a man to Room B and return to the booth, take a seat, and am about to resume seating chart updates when I see him.

A young guy in street clothes craning over his phone, as the other hand pushes a lightweight aluminum gurney bearing nothing but a flat black bag, a body bag heading in the direction of the ICU. It passes within feet of the booth where I gawk.

I've never seen an empty body bag before, or a filled one. Empty, it looks no more consequential than a garment bag for a nice suit.

Once, in a telehealth setting, it would have been my job to discharge the deceased individual down the hall not to HOME but to DEATH in the program called eCare Manager. To do it I had to get an accurate time of death—down to the minute—from the nurse here. If the nurse did not call with it, I had to call the nurse and ask. There was always a lag between the death and the recording, twenty or thirty minutes of electronic limbo. Trying to make the process feel more humane, I had that habit of looking up the patient's age and full name during the wait, but it did not much help alter the vibe of callousness. Bright sophisticated screens were very good at taking the uniqueness out of a life, reducing it to fields of data that all looked the same.

Twenty minutes later the dead patient passes by, pushed hearseward by phone-tapping remover. The body bag is flatter than I would have imagined. A ceremonial purple cloth has been spread over the top. The gurney creeps because the unsuspecting drug-peddling robot is just ahead, moving at the programmed methodical speed. At last the quixotic procession rolls out of view.

COVID? OD? Stroke? Bullet? Teenager? Truck driver? Entrepreneur? The eICU manager told me that 80 percent of ICU patients actually die of septic shock that can be caused by many maladies that stop major organs from functioning.

Was the remover playing a video game? Seeking news updates? The internet is like the dazzling sun at La Jolla beach. The force to go to and go to until there is nothing left but lying beside it . . . swimming in it . . . continual splashes of energy obscuring all that is not it.

I stand in the booth. I reach for the stars. I fail to touch the ceiling. I step out of the booth and head toward the men's room. Next to the door is a bank of staff elevators. The sidestepping remover is trying to fit the gurney into a car and struggling—half in, half out. . . .

It's a funny restroom. The gooseneck tap is equipped with an electric eye. The eye is supposed to trigger a flow of water when hands are in view, but the eye needs a monocle. It does not work. The first two shifts I waved hands like a philharmonic conductor and not a drop. The gestures—driven by pandemic hygiene desperation—finally got so elaborate that I accidently smacked the tap, and it rocked in a loose base, and water flowed. I throttle the silly goose again. Water sluices over hands. I wet a paper towel, shove it under masks.

There is a justice in this. Justice that an eICU discharger to DEATH should finally have to see the real thing swing by his desk. Justice, but god it is sad.

Room A is empty. Room B is empty. I strip off the door labels. Then the phone rings and I scurry and A is occupied again. Returning to the booth I reread a note taped to the bottom of one Plexiglas panel: "Where did my little owl buddy go? Please return. Volunteer Deena." The owl: symbol of wisdom in Greece. Yes, please promptly return.

Phone in my backpack dings. It's got to be Ivan sending more links to glorious music via What's App. Aretha. Gil Scott-Heron. Activist Ivan, in his apartment on Featherbed Lane in the Bronx, peels green peppers so as not to ingest factory wax the vegetables are coated with.

Phone rings.

"Need a consult room for the family of Izzy."

"Okay—I'll give you B."

The nurse thanks me like some do. The usual. I hear nothing awry.

I exit the booth, and call out the patient's first name twice. The second time the spouse hears, lowers phone, grabs a jacket off the chair next to hers. She is short and broad shouldered. Into the B door slot I slide the label. I flick on the room light.

"Make yourself comfortable. If you'd like to close the door, go ahead."

She's on her phone again and doesn't respond. I've been back at the booth for a few minutes when I glance over and see the door is now shut. She did hear. Five minutes after that two men in scrubs approach the door, slow, and look at each other as if wordlessly debating entry order. I know the surgeon's name from the eICU data-entry days but I've never seen Towers. Which is he? Once when a nurse here called to warn the eICU of an incoming "hot mess on a copter," she added a terse: "Towers knows."

The clinicians finish their jig and enter. Door clicks shut.

Right after that, I see a huddle of nurses in flamboyant OR headwraps (butterflies, NFL insignias) beside a hall wall. Their gazes are pinned on the door of consult Room B.

Then it comes. An explosion of grief from in there. Screams, mixed up with words I can't make out, build to an initial scorching peak, subside for a minute, build again in thick hot volume. Izzy was forty-nine years old. In for a back operation. Phone rings. I pick up.

"We've just had a death in the OR. Please direct chaplaincy to the consult room."

Before I can respond the nurse hangs up.

We've just had a death in the OR.

I've just—like a dockhand on the levee Lethe—delivered a stranger to the room where she has been informed her husband is dead. In Room C still sits the new mother, storing nourishment for her infant as a soundtrack of loss pours down halls, through a waiting room of faces now not turning at the slightest sound but staring down.

"Where is the family?"

The badge pinned to the plaid dress-shirt pocket reads Rev. Theo. He's got a broad chin and an Air Force crew cut. He wears wire rims, grips a Bible.

"In . . . B. One person . . . the spouse . . . doctors are with her."

He nods. I thank him for coming. He nods again. We stand wordless, on opposite sides of Plexiglas, until the doctors exit the room where the widow still sobs. Theo enters.

Nurses surround the doctors in the hall. I see DONE written across Izzy's data on the procedure list. I don't recall scribbling the letters. It is what I usually write after a family has been successfully reunited with their loved one.

"I think I know where we can put the body," pipes a nurse.

"You do?" asks one of the doctors, the dark-haired one. Is it Towers?

"The room is empty now but it might not be for long."

"Good," says the doctor with less hair. "I can help you with that."

"I think we can take care of it," says another nurse.

Exit RNs to deal with corpse. Exit doctors. Exit the young mother from Room C. She wears a startled expression as she reinhabits her spot in the hushed waiting room.

The door to Room B opens. Theo walks the widow to the elevator. She is on her phone: "turned him on his back and. . . ." After she enters the car he approaches the booth.

"She's going out to smoke."

"Ah."

"More family will be coming, Ben. I need a place to meet with them."

Theo is standing no less straight than before and his voice is even. A leader.

"Uh . . . let me see. I'll ask the registrars."

I hurry back there. Only one dueling banjo is present now, and she really picks a jarring tune this time. There is, she indicates, *no place whatsoever up here* set aside for chaplaincy to meet with families. I give her a five-bar bluesy glare.

Hasn't this happened before? It has to have happened before. And there's no protocol to ensure a grieving family's privacy? Nor a set venue for OR corpse storage? I'll be winging this like the others? Oh yeah, a slipper and slider exactly like the rest.

"Let's uh . . ." I say to Theo not knowing what I am going to say next, but a plan does stumble into place. I assign him Room C to meet with family as long as necessary—the room farthest from Room A, the most commonly used consult space. I walk him to the door. The young mother left the light on. The IN USE sign is still in the door slot. I wish him luck.

"Thank you, Ben. They are going to be loud."

For the first time I hear dread chipping at the edges of his solid enunciation. He and the Bible enter. He leaves the door open a crack. I return to the Kafka booth, and sit, and don't have time to wonder *what next?* One of the doctors that broke the bad news reappears. Hands on hips. Mask below chin. Stubble. His eyes are an enigmatic brown.

"Where's the rest of the family?"

"Not here yet."

"Hey, I've got another surgery to get ready for."

List indicates it is a lap-sleeve gastrectomy on morbidly obese Dakotan.

"Want me to call you when more family arrive?"

"Do that. Dr. Towers. Mike Towers. My number is. . . ."

Outside, as she smokes in front of the hospital's main entrance, the widow has been making calls, instructing relatives to go to the second floor where I sit. I want to run away by now. I do not run this time. Someone has to be here to direct family members to Theo. They arrive singly and in pairs. In shock, none are wearing masks. I don't have the heart (or is it the professionalism?) to hassle them. In a voice that doesn't sound to me much like my voice, I say, "Sorry for your loss," as I lead mourners to the solace of the gospel.

The one who really gets me is the wiry man with the close-cropped reddish beard, orange construction vest. Face grooved with solemnity. The Van Gogh hollows for cheeks. There he was, working on an outdoor project on a frigid day, when the cell phone rang. . . .

Widow returns, enters C. I hear no more sobbing, no more screams. It is a quieter room than Rev. Theo expected. I call Towers as he requested.

"Mike," he answers quick.

"This is the surgery waiting host. The family of Izzy has arrived."

"Let me talk to them," he commands.

"I . . . can't."

"You can't?"

"The phone I'm holding is like a phone in an old motel. I can't pick it up and carry it across the hall to the consult room. The cord isn't long enough."

He makes a noise as if he has never heard of any such thing as a landline. Dial tone.

I exit the booth with swerving steps, keeping my back to the waiting room. I've given up on seating chart accuracy today. The hell with more arrows.

"Will you notify the family the body is in room 2208?"

I turn. It's a nurse in the hall. I don't know her. I step back. She's under pressure. How you react to pressure tells the most about who you are. Few function perfectly.

"Will you do that for me? Tell the family. . . ."

I worry masks as if they are a beard to tug when confused.

"Don't you think . . . a clinician should be the one to do that?"

"Oh, right. I'll do it then."

"Try Room C."

She pivots, leans in, passes along corpse location, runs down the hall.

Phone rings. I get to the booth in time to take the call. Consult room needed for family of Lyle. I put them in A. Phone rings again. Consult room needed for family of Coreen. I put them in B. Nothing extraordinary about any of these actions, but after the OR death all movement feels abnormal, off, and out of control. The Prairie Center unit I work for has spoiled me. Plenty of staff. Well organized. Most patients in and out fast, under their own power.

I stick a straw under the beard, sip water. A break, I think, and just then, up the hall glides another gurney with a flat dark bag on it, pushed by a different remover in street clothes. He's not mastering a video game. He's looking where he's going, and he's going to the ICU where another patient has perished. Six Dakotans die of COVID on this day.

Through the cracked door of consulting Room A wafts a surgeon's merry baritone: "Full of hair and fatty tissue. No cancer. Happy New Year."

When remover returns, headed toward a dance with a staff elevator car, the bag full of remains is not draped in ceremonial purple. Maybe the family couldn't afford the perk?

I think of the soft-spoken Lakota Nation member named Nelson who spent time with me in the lobby recently. He told about getting drafted by the Army in the late 1960s. When he and a friend, also drafted, reported to the induction site, there was a big surprise. An officer told Nelson he was more needed on the home front because of his good grades. Nelson applied to UC Berkeley the next month, graduating in four years with a degree in water management. He does that work to this day on the Pine Ridge Reservation. His friend was killed by a sniper six hours after arriving in Vietnam. The story haunted Nelson, now was trailing me. Because you don't get A's you are more expendable at age eighteen? Anyone who sees the dead knows the luck of living, but the dead can't tell you what they've discovered, no matter how close you were to them in life. The quiet of voices you can't hear is deafening.

"How are you, Ben?"

It's Pam again, plastic bonnet and bloodshot eyes.

"Someone died on the table, two others in the ICU," I whisper.

"You don't say?" she mutters, head gyrating.

I hear a pack of cigarettes in her sentences now. Spending so much time in the halls here, she's probably seen hundreds of body bags wheeling in and out during the pandemic.

"I can't wait to get back to the Prairie Center."

"Don't blame you. Hang in."

"You too."

When the hanging is finally finished, as I'm reaching for my unlucky blue sweater, Rev. Theo appears on the other side of the booth.

"I don't need the room anymore, Ben."

"Thanks for telling me."

I crumple the note—*C in use as a mourning room*—written for the next host.

"And thanks, Ben, for your help today."

"Is this your only job?"

"I have a church. I'm here part-time."

He leaves. The young mother approaches.

"I need to pump again."

"No problem. Use B this time."

I can't chance exposing her to lingering exhalations of unmasked mourners.

I jot a new note for the next host—*B in use as mother's room*—and look out for volunteer Deena, my jacket on, but she does not show.

Has the search for her owl buddy taken her to the Adirondacks? After three calls I learn she called in sick to Judith the volunteer coordinator. I am told to arrange for backup on my own by dialing the ambulatory unit. I do. A patient care technician materializes. Polite Paul in mint-green scrubs. I apologize for the state of the seating chart. He shrugs, says: "Well, I see you have phone numbers for everyone, that's the important thing."

I drive to the aquatic center. In the lap lane, before reaching the wall, I flip on my back, dip head under, gaze up through the water at the steely glare of the ceiling lights.

December 31
"Life-Flighted in from Le Mars"

As I make coffee, the pugilistic diction of Paul James on 1010 WINS reports that the most googled search term in 2021 is the name of would-be social media star and confirmed murderer Brian Laundrie. Yesterday almost half a million COVID cases were tallied. Seven days ago South Dakota became the last state to verify a first case of the Omicron variant.

I bring Anne's coffee up to her, a ritual to cherish because it is so straightforward and always makes her smile under covers.

I enter into the cold after checking to see the street is clear of rough customers. Fourteen degrees. The garage door is nice and shuts after only six tries. That inspires me to wish it a Happy New Year.

Today can't be worse than yesterday? Yesterday, upon arriving home from the aquatic center, I knocked a jar of salsa off a storage shelf and it shattered, sending the red stuff flying. Lurid smears on shelves, on the wall, on wine bottles, on the unfinished floor.

The concierge at the hospital's main entrance, perched on a stool, is wearing a conical green HAPPY 2022 cap. To the right are the staff elevators. To the left is the cafeteria. The food line is closed. Nobody is there. I divert. I stall. I don't want to enter the Kafka booth yet. I walk to a table next to a window, chew on air purified by my masks, and stare out at the dawn of the end of 2021, calculating gains and losses, feeling a glissando of urgency to make more progress in many areas—economic, therapeutic, artistic.

When I finally reach the surgery waiting area I find it empty.

HAPPY NEW YEAR (pink letters outlined in blue) is printed at the top of the surgery list on the desk in the Kafka booth. One patient is having a leg amputated due to diabetic gangrene. Three thumb amputations. A "foreign body" needs to be removed from a child. A man who fell seven feet will have back surgery. An EtOH—severe abuser of alcohol—needs a facial laceration repaired. That abbreviation, EtOH, I frequently entered as an eICU diagnosis when admitting patients who had poisoned themselves in local alleys.

I unlock the consult rooms, let dueling banjos know I am on duty. Apparently they are competing to see who can wear the reddest red. It is a draw. After we enact the scantest of exchanges they resume trading words of false merriment that hurt to hear.

Hall traffic is sporadic. A nurse in a COVID-proof papper—sci-fi helmet and breathing tank. The buzzing pill-pushing robot. The intercom prays: "Lord, as we come to the end of this year of grace you have given us. . . ." The first people to check in are women of different generations. Their loved one is having a complex C-section operation scheduled to last eight hours. They settle down for the long haul against a far wall.

"Hi, Ben!"

"Amber!"

She stands in the hall next to the booth. Her high-pitched voice is scratchier than usual. She is wearing the food-service black smock and matching pants.

"So glad to see you! Where have you been?"

"I was recovering from surgery."

She pulls down the smock collar. It looks like her neck has been struck by a sword. The scar is more than six inches long and jagged with stitches.

"Thyroid cancer. It's spread into my chest, they tell me. I'll be operated on again next week. Doesn't hurt though. I came in to train the replacement for my next leave."

She pulls up and tidies the smock collar. Festive fingernail polish.

"I'm so sorry."

"Oh well. How's Anne?"

"She's fine."

"Give her my regards."

"I will."

"Have to go now! Have a good day."

Could anyone replace Amber? The pale scrawny kid who is going to try now stands behind her, wearing a black skullcap to match the smock and pants. Throughout the shift, they'll pass and I'll hear Amber, possibly dying Amber, patiently instructing him on nuances of tray management. Thoughtful loyal being. I'll need to tell Anne the news of her ordeal.

Digit amputation candidates, and family members, arrive simultaneously. The patient that cannot be checked in immediately is sent by a dueling banjo to the waiting room, where he is immediately approached by a functionary in scrubs who loudly explains the importance of declaring whether or not ownership of the severed tissue will be relinquished. There is a form. The form is handed over. Befuddled patient pinches the form, looking up as if asking his maker about the possible uses of a severed thumb . . . then signs.

Elevator keeps opening. I chirp my tune. Seating chart fills. It's not as placid as I hoped: *camo shirt / pink pullover / couple, young / Vikings hoodie / canary yellow hoodie / black jacket / red flannel fleece / bright blue hoodie / brown cap / Lake Okoboji T-shirt. . . .*

"You're working today, Ben?!"

Familiar timbre of nicotine and pandemic weariness: Pam under the crinkly cap.

"And you too!"

"No way around it."

"Isn't that the truth."

"What can we do?"

"Exactly. Happy 2022. Make it new, Pam!"

Puppets of her cheeks waltz again above the mask secluding her cynical smile.

"Make it new? Oh, I don't know about that."

She moves on. I wonder again what went wrong for Towers in the OR yesterday. Where is the family of Izzy today? Waiting room occupants swig lattes. Talk sports. Sail the sea of the internet. Not a pacer in the bunch, thank goodness.

Phone rings. First consult room request. I lead family to Room A. Surgeon bellows news as he enters: "A very good salvage procedure!" More room requests follow.

Today's surgeries, save for the C-section, are short. I'm up and down for more than an hour, with a few quick coffee-caused trips to the restroom where I throttle the silly goose of a tap to make it work. Why hasn't the defect been addressed? By midmorning the waiting room is almost empty, save for the C-section vigil, and a lady with dark curly hair reading a Grisham novel, waiting for news about her husband's port placement.

I think of Marion, the best boss I ever had. She liked to hire striving artists to do clerical work for the *World News Digest*, a mainstay publication of the reference publisher Facts On File. One year Marion went so far as to arrange a variety show at the Bowery Poetry Club to showcase our diverse projects. I think of the evening I read a poem called "The Bird Buriers" in the circular room that had been the first surgical arena of Bellevue Hospital before becoming a cafeteria decorated with a still existent WPA mural depicting a cow-milking facility, among other 1930s food-production images. I think of Brooklyn-bred Richard, a former coworker at FOF, who never forgets to call on my birthday.

When Anne and I moved here to further our study, in situ, of the Midwest that deeply affected our childhoods in very different ways, he was stunned: "But Ben . . . when I think of what a New Yorker is . . . that's you!" That's who I built atop the mud and the rust. A peculiar hybrid, another floater. Being claimed by two worlds meant belonging fully to none. That creates alternatives. Makes you want to build bridges and cross them.

Three masked individuals stutter-step toward the booth. They look lost. They look in trouble. Young woman in a pink hoodie. Middle-aged man in an Iowa Hawkeye hoodie. Middle-aged woman wearing a down coat. She speaks.

"Our son-in-law was just life-flighted in from Le Mars."

Le Mars, Iowa. Home of the Blue Bunny Ice Cream parlor and Archie's Waeside, a steak house. The birthplace of my father's mother Rose, Catholic wearer of white gloves.

By car this trio followed the Eurocopter H145 that lifted off from the small hospital there.

"Can you tell us what room Walt is in?"

"I—has he arrived yet?"

"Our daughter texted that the helicopter landed."

He could have gone straight into surgery. If not there, the ICU.

"For privacy reasons I have no access to patient room assignments. But there are staff members nearby who do. I'll check with them. Wait here."

Dueling banjos are gone. Starting the party early. Gone. What now? Their dumb seasonal decorations offer no clue. Le Mars eyes gauge my approach for meaning.

"The registrars have left for the day. The best thing might be to ask downstairs."

"The person in the lobby sent us up here."

"Then, well . . . let's. . . ."

The man blinks slowly. The two women look puzzled for good reason.

"I'll escort you to the entrance of the ICU. There you can call in and see if a room has been assigned yet. How does that sound?"

"We appreciate your help," says the man softly.

I lead them past the consult rooms and a long row of windows. I turn left, they turn left. Ahead are the doors to vented COVID patients and other critical situations.

Doors are locked for safety reasons. There have been cases in the urban Midwest of a gang member visiting an ICU to finish off a rival. Once in this unit brass knuckles tumbled from a patient's backpack when the nurse picked it up.

The woman in the coat calls in. She is told Walt has not arrived but that a room has been assigned. She says the number out loud. I write the number down.

"She told us to go to the ICU waiting room and they'll let us know when he gets there. Oh . . . I forgot the number already."

I give it to her. We follow wall arrows to the ICU Family Waiting Room around the corner. The door is locked. Fuck.

"I apologize. Huh. I know. Let's . . . let's go back the way we came. There is a spot near the vending machines where you can wait for now."

It's one of those mile-long short walks. We pass panes displaying the haze of the year's last day. The silence is awful but worse would be to break it in the wrong way.

I recall a nurse's story about a party thrown to celebrate this new ICU, execs raising toasts to a place that would treat addicts dying of cirrhosis of the liver. Obviously it has no dedicated elevator to make the exit of the dead more private, dignified. There are doctors here who also find it odd the ICU exists on the second floor and not nearer to the ER. Like many ICUs it contains a room with bulletproof windows to protect an ill visiting dignitary.

Is Carrie in the ICU today? She's another nurse who soon figured out the actual unit was preferable to the frustrating technosnarl of virtual care. She'd be of help if she was on duty. She was easy to work with and fair. She liked lakes, like me.

At the booth we turn left and soon reach the cola machines, couches, tables.

"My daughter should be coming soon," says the younger woman.

"She's texted that she's with Walt," says the older woman.

"I'll be on the lookout. I'll point her back here. What's her name?"

"Mary."

As I walk back to my station, I realize I did not see one other hospital employee on duty between here and the ICU. The void extends to the abandoned registrar area, all the way to the doors of the Post-/Pre-Op unit. How could this be allowed for even ten minutes? I always take many notes when I am trained, but in this case I was tutored for two full days by a Belinda who never mentioned mother's rooms or life-flight situations or deaths in the OR or chaplains lacking facilities. She discussed exciting topics such as the day's cafeteria offerings, her son the lawyer, and which side of Maui is the correct side to stay on during a December vacation. She is there right now, toes in the water. I wish a jellyfish on her.

I enter the booth. I shut my eyes, try to slow things way down, channeling the piano stylings of Bill Evans on *Sunday at the Village Vanguard*. His playing is like listening to a candle flicker, each note a drop of wax, the sound of incandescence. . . .

"Want a Dew? The expiration date is only the twentieth."

Finally another face! Not the one I need, but familiar. The uniformed delivery man tormented by waste. Poor guy, he also has a position perfectly unsuited to his disposition.

"Thanks, but not today."

He pushes onward toward the next dubious harvest of drinkable cola as a very young ICU nurse approaches.

"Did the family get settled?" he asks.

"They did. What happened to the ICU waiting room?"

"It got canceled."

Canceled? I don't have time to ask him to explain. He's gone.

A chaplain in a V-neck sweater and slacks—not Theo—steps up to bat next, wanting to know where the family of Walt is. I point. Then in front of me is a KC Chiefs hoodie, blond hair.

"Are you Mary?"

She is. I lead her to the vending machine area where she is hugged. I turn around, spying a volunteer wheeling a patient down the hall toward the abandoned registrar's area. Volunteers were given the day off, but Mack reported anyway. Minutes later he's back at the elevator, telling the patient: "One thing I can't do, fella, is leave you up here stranded. I'll take you back downstairs and talk to the gal down there about what we should do."

A bustle in the hall. Walt on the gurney equipped with an IV and extra apparatus. The chaplain following, and the fatigued Le Mars family, one two three four.

I and my headache enter the booth. Hour and a half left. Maybe I should have trusted the first vision for how to earn a living in this idiosyncratic state. Like the best inspirations, it came out of nowhere—the concept of selling McCann's steel-cut oatmeal ("Brown sugar? Butter? Half-and-half? Raisins?") from a downtown cart shaped like the can those Irish oats are imported in. There's that left to try. Or a school of the visual arts. Never been. Pratt?

Phone rings. A room number for the port placement patient. I lead the wife back there. She praises the plots of the novels of Grisham. That leaves only two women sitting where they have been since 7:00 a.m. Right before the end of the shift I visit them.

"Good luck."

"Thanks. We just heard they finished with the front," one says. She points to her phone and the EASE surgery tracking app.

"Great to hear."

My replacement is on time. Paul again. Saint Paul. I wish him a happy holiday.

I sling the backpack over my shoulder, and on the elevator lean against the steel wall of the car. It's New Year's Day tomorrow, and I leave behind a precarious birth in progress. Baby New Year arriving with few assurances as the aged year is just about to expire.

January 2022
The Rongeur

Back in the Prairie Center for the first time this month, at a frigid predawn windy garbage-bin-rolling hour! WKCR's Daybreak Express jazz show fills the lobby with the muscular sax sound of Illinois Jacquet, a player famous for his solo on "Flying Home."

I flick on desk lamp, resupply mask table, place in a corner the yellow CAUTION sign the night cleaning person always leaves standing in the middle of the floor after mopping. The surgery list is not long—the December volume prompted by insurance-deductible considerations is over. After setting up, like a primal creature I gaze into the darkness waiting for the sun to rise. Each shift is an evolution rerun. The night makes the cold feel colder, as some awful poet must have written. Maybe I wrote that once. Probably.

Today, the fifth, more than 800,000 Americans will test positive for the COVID virus. Tomorrow is the ninetieth birthday of Dick the volunteer, who bakes chocolate cakes for the other volunteers and, when not delivering flowers, patrols the extensive plantings at the Prairie Center, removing trash from enormous pots shaped like Rocky Mountain boulders. Sometimes he crawls into those pots. Recently he told me a funny thing: he served in the navy nowhere near water, at an ordnance station in the Mojave Desert.

Zero degrees outside and it is cold in the lobby. Broken foyer ceiling heaters are not blasting warmth. Each time sliding doors open a new current of arctic air is sucked in. The air flows toward the desk and stops and pools. Paralytic molecules. I have five layers on. I wear the tall fur hat with earflaps that makes me look like a guard at Buckingham Palace. One arriving radiologist bursts out laughing under his mask. Others are concerned. I point at the fur hat: "It's like having a radiator strapped to my head."

Bundled nurses exclaim, "Holy buckets, it's cold!" or "Oh my stars, it's cold!" or "Uff da!"

"Welcome to Ice Station Zebra," I say, or "Congratulations, you made it across the tundra" or "I'm starting to wonder if Shackleton will stumble in and ask directions."

He doesn't but Joel does. My erudite friend who drives for Wheelchair Express. We don't have time to talk, but set up a call. He makes a mean old-fashioned. Thanks to consistent precautions he still hasn't caught the virus. Ought to be a Hall of Fame for that.

Minnesota father's tale: "My son told me he was going to a New Year's Eve party at Duffy's, and I told him that if he did he'd have to quarantine for fourteen days before seeing me again. He said 'Oh, Dad' but didn't go."

Retired schoolteacher's tale: "My son refused to get vaccinated. He got the virus. Then he took his family on a vacation to Jamaica and got it again. He couldn't fly back with them. And the rest of the family, when they landed, tested positive."

It's been the same story for months. Tellers are inevitably bewildered and/or anguished. To be incapable of uniting to deal with an epidemic points to a painful, dizzying phenomenon: concepts of family, and of country, are so widely varied from individual to individual that often the outcome is indecipherability on all levels of the social unit—smallest to largest. How do you receive, let alone follow, orders from entities you fail to understand? That do not talk your language? Long claws of crisis have ripped to bits the tissue paper of rhetoric that fostered fragile notions of compatibility. Does that partially explain the toilet-paper run early on? A spot-on instinct that tissue is about all we have to work with to hold things together? So gather ye a thousand rolls! Don't be glum! Get to work! Re-create the crepe illusion! The tellers of these tales rarely hit a note of surrender. They are hardly giving up. They want things to be as they thought they were. For human reasons, they pray for a debunking of the debunking.

Hey, I know the feeling—I had it at age twelve, staring out a torn window screen at a city that could seem to consist of thousands of citizens with a talent for wishing away dumps like ours, overgrown with crisis. I resented them, but really I did not blame them past a certain point. I didn't want my life—the crap scattered everywhere in that room—to be true. If it was, there'd be no cleaning it up. If it was, there'd be dirt in my teeth for the rest of my life. . . .

The big problem today is how to explain to the boss who set up the Main OR gig why it did not work out for me. Nicely, I get the task out of the way early.

"Too rugged for me over there, Lynnette. I haven't the constitution of a nurse. I'm more of a clamshell that never completely closes. I tend to absorb too much."

She listens well, nodding, then thinks out loud.

"There's so much to do here—and you get along so well with everyone—seems to me we'll probably be able to find you five extra hours on most weeks. Guiding patients to rooms after they check in upstairs. Or putting together information packets."

"Fine with me."

I had the qualifications. It's how I started the whole day-job saga in 1986, collating international-economic-conference packets at the New York Stock Exchange, in the regal boardroom where the rulers were to assemble. It was decorated with oils of scions like J. P. Morgan. In a corner, a priceless gift from Iran's shah. We were a team of four hungry graduate students stuffing folders after dark. The task was overseen by the Exchange's general counsel James Buck in his contrived summer boater, red bowtie, vest, *and* watch chain. He sent us home in limos. Mine whizzed up Sixth Avenue, stopping at West Fourth, a short walk from my corner of a shared studio apartment where I slept on a foam-rubber slab on the floor next to a transistor radio tuned to WQXR and Nimet.

"Good, Ben. We'll see if we can't get that going then."

Later that morning, three events occur that I marvel at for the rest of the month as I pull successive shifts in the lobby and add others on the fourth floor, where, as promised, I am put to work at a rostrum facing a window overlooking the parking lot and the surrounding neighborhood, where, in front of one bungalow, an American flag flies upside down.

It's tranquil finger work, compiling glossy copies of *A Patient's Guide to a Successful Recovery* with four black-and-white forms. Paper clip on side, add to stack, begin again—paper clip on side, add to stack, begin again—paper clip on side, add to stack, begin again. . . . I'm not bored. To me the core of being a writer is the willingness to start over. It's never a negative thing. It's an occasion for renewal.

And as I collate and collate, I cogitate on the carnival of the first 2022 shift in the lobby. Who could have predicted any of it?

First, a nurse named Wally steps off the elevator holding a UPS box from a medical supply company addressed to Ben P. Miller at the main hospital. I tell him I haven't ordered anything sent here. He replies that I am the only Ben P. Miller on the campus, directs me to open the box, make absolutely sure the contents are not mine, and he'll take care of the rest, send the package back to the company. I pry open the cardboard. Inside is a medical instrument resembling a long pair of pliers crossed with a vise and a fish scaler. He says it is a "rongeur" used to chew through a skull to expose the brain so lobes can be operated on. We laugh about the bizarre mistake. He takes the box away. I don't get it. Then I do? *The pen I've been keeping pandemic logs with is a kind of rongeur! A precision tool designed to reach the place where ideas thrive, memories shelter.*

About an hour later, a sedan pulls up outside the foyer, and I tug on gloves and go out and ask the driver if a wheelchair is needed. He nods. It is for his mother, sitting next to him. She is ninety, according to the surgery list. I wheel the chair out to the curb, next to the passenger-side door, and the son takes over in the extreme cold. He opens the door. He leans between the wheelchair and the figure clad in pinkish layers down to her slippers. "Put your arm around my neck, Mom," he murmurs until she does. "Now, Mom, hold tight. . . ." He's half in the car—this guy wearing just a Sportz Bar cap, jeans, unzipped jacket. He lifts her off the car seat while reaching back and down to scoop up her frail legs. She moans a good question, "Why does it have to be so cold?" He turns with her in his arms. He incrementally lowers her into the chair as I watch. I see, at last, how to do it— how a forbearing and loving son picks up a broken parent, when the pieces are large enough to be embraced.

In the last hour an ambulance arrives from Phillips, Minnesota. Two EMTs open the back door and slide out a yellow gurney. It emerges flat, the patient hooked to an IV, unshaven and appearing to be made of not much more than sheets that wrap him. EMTs do not address the patient. I wonder if he is in a coma. They make the gurney grow, rise, expanding the Xs underneath, and the pair push the still man through swooshing sliding doors to where I stand, arm extending into the elevator car to keep the door from closing. I tell EMTs to take their time. EMTs briefly discuss how to edge in the bulky conveyance and go to work. They slide the gurney a little this way, a little that way. The patient's eyes have flicked open: he's not in a coma. Gurney inches forward into the elevator car. I'm looking at the patient's pale eyes and pale skin. He's looking up. If he was looking at me we'd be almost face-to-face since the bed is so high, and I find I cannot let him pass unacknowledged. He's come far. He's been aware the whole trip, just lying there, transported in the bubble of his disease. That isolation strikes me as unacceptable. "Hi, John," I say. And without missing a beat, in a voice that is clear and far stronger than he looks, a voice that addresses me head-on though he is still looking straight up, a voice cello-like and elaborate with vibrato, he replies: "Helloooo." Speaks as if he is not ill and I am not in my awkward position—as if we both have, for an instant, outwitted the labyrinth.

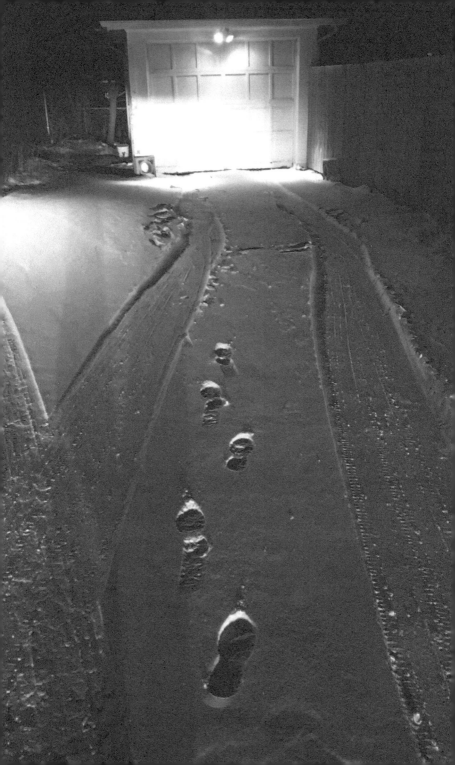

ACKNOWLEDGMENTS

I owe gratitude to the unforgettable John A. Williams, a model of artistry and fortitude who continues to inform my practice daily. I also want to express my appreciation for the extraordinary support I have received over the years from Dorothy James, Larry Ling, Wes and Patti Pierson, Stephanie Volmer, and Gail and Jim Wiese. Finally, it is important to recognize Jackson Lears, Karen Parker Lears, and Ginger Thompson for professional encouragement at various vital junctures in the development of this particular form.

ABOUT THE AUTHOR

BEN MILLER is the author of *River Bend Chronicle: The Junkification of a Boyhood Idyll amid the Curious Glory of Urban Iowa*. He has published in *Raritan, Salmagundi, One Story, The Georgia Review, Inscription, New England Review*, and *Best American Experimental Writing*. His essays have been reprinted or noted nine times in *Best American Essays*. His awards include fellowships from the National Endowment for the Arts and the Radcliffe Institute, as well as grants from the South Dakota Arts Council and the Schlesinger Library on the History of Women in America. He has been a finalist for the Bellwether Prize for Socially Engaged Fiction.